OSTEOPOROSIS DIET COOKBOOK FOR SENIORS

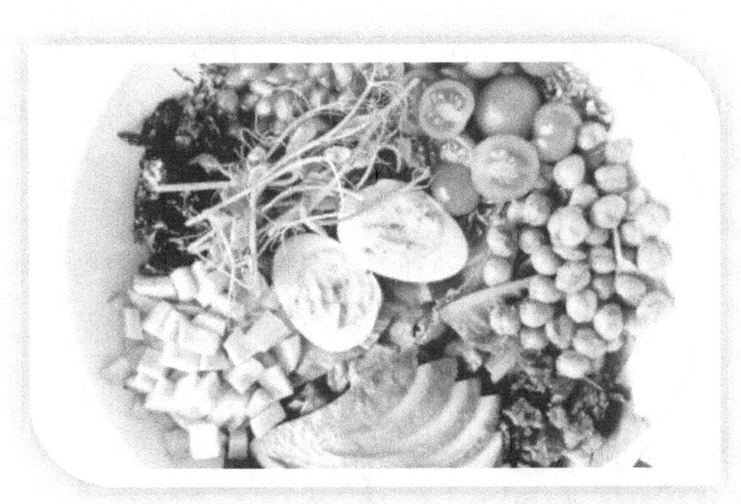

The comprehensive science-backed osteoporosis nutrition guide with bone-healthy recipes for older people

Dr. Linda Thompson

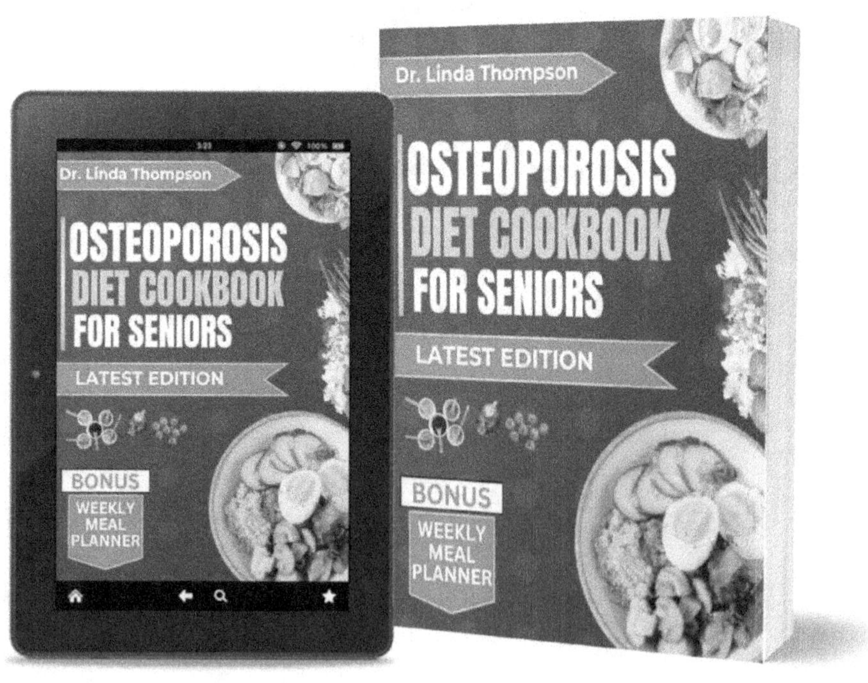
Dr. Linda Thompson
OSTEOPOROSIS
DIET COOKBOOK
FOR SENIORS
LATEST EDITION
BONUS
WEEKLY
MEAL
PLANNER
Dr. Linda Thompson
OSTEOPOROSIS
DIET COOKBOOK
FOR SENIORS
LATEST EDITION
BONUS
WEEKLY
MEAL
PLANNER

TABLE OF CONTENTS

OSTEOPOROSIS
Healthy bone
Osteoporosis

Welcome to a journey towards stronger, healthier bones. As an orthopedist with years of experience, I have witnessed firsthand the profound impact that osteoporosis can have on the lives of seniors. It is a silent thief, stealthily robbing individuals of their independence and vitality. Yet, amidst this challenge lies an empowering truth: through the transformative power of nutrition and lifestyle choices, we can fortify our bones and reclaim our well-being.

I am deeply honored to embark on this journey with you—a journey that not only delves into the depths of osteoporosis but also empowers you to take charge of your bone health through the transformative power of nutrition.

Allow me to share a heartfelt story— a story that embodies the essence of our mission within these pages. Meet Victoria, a remarkable woman whose resilience and determination inspired the creation of this cookbook. Victoria, my beloved sister, faced the daunting challenge of osteoporosis in her later years. Witnessing her struggle firsthand ignited a passion within me to explore innovative ways to combat this silent yet debilitating condition.

Victoria's journey was not without its hurdles. The fractures, the pain, the moments of uncertainty—each obstacle seemed insurmountable. However, amidst the shadows of despair, a beacon of hope emerged. Through meticulous research, compassionate care, and unwavering support, I guided Victoria on a path towards healing—one rooted in the fundamental principles of nutrition and holistic wellness.

Together, we embarked on a transformative journey—one that celebrated the innate healing potential of wholesome, nutrient-rich foods. From vibrant salads bursting with leafy greens to nourishing soups brimming with bone-strengthening minerals, each meal became a testament to Victoria's resilience and determination. With each bite, she nourished not only her body but also her spirit—a poignant reminder of the profound connection between food and healing.

And as the days turned into weeks, and the weeks into months, Victoria's progress was nothing short of miraculous. The fractures healed, the pain subsided, and a newfound vitality radiated from within. Through the power of nutrition, Victoria defied the odds, emerging stronger and more resilient than ever before.

Inspired by Victoria's remarkable journey, I embarked on a mission—to share the invaluable lessons learned, the delicious recipes crafted, and the transformative insights gained. Within the pages of this cookbook, you will find more than just recipes—you will find a roadmap to vibrant health, a blueprint for reclaiming your vitality, and a source of inspiration to embark on your own journey towards osteoporosis prevention and management.

In this cookbook, I invite you to join me on a voyage of discovery—a journey that transcends mere recipes and transcends into the realm of healing. Here, you will find not just a collection of culinary delights, but a comprehensive guide infused with scientific wisdom and practical advice. Together, we will unravel the mysteries of osteoporosis, understanding its nuances, its challenges, and its conquerable nature.

So, dear reader, I invite you to join me on this extraordinary adventure—a journey of healing, hope, and culinary delight. Together, let us nourish our bones, nurture our bodies, and embrace the boundless potential of optimal health.

With warmest regards,

[Dr. Linda Thompson]

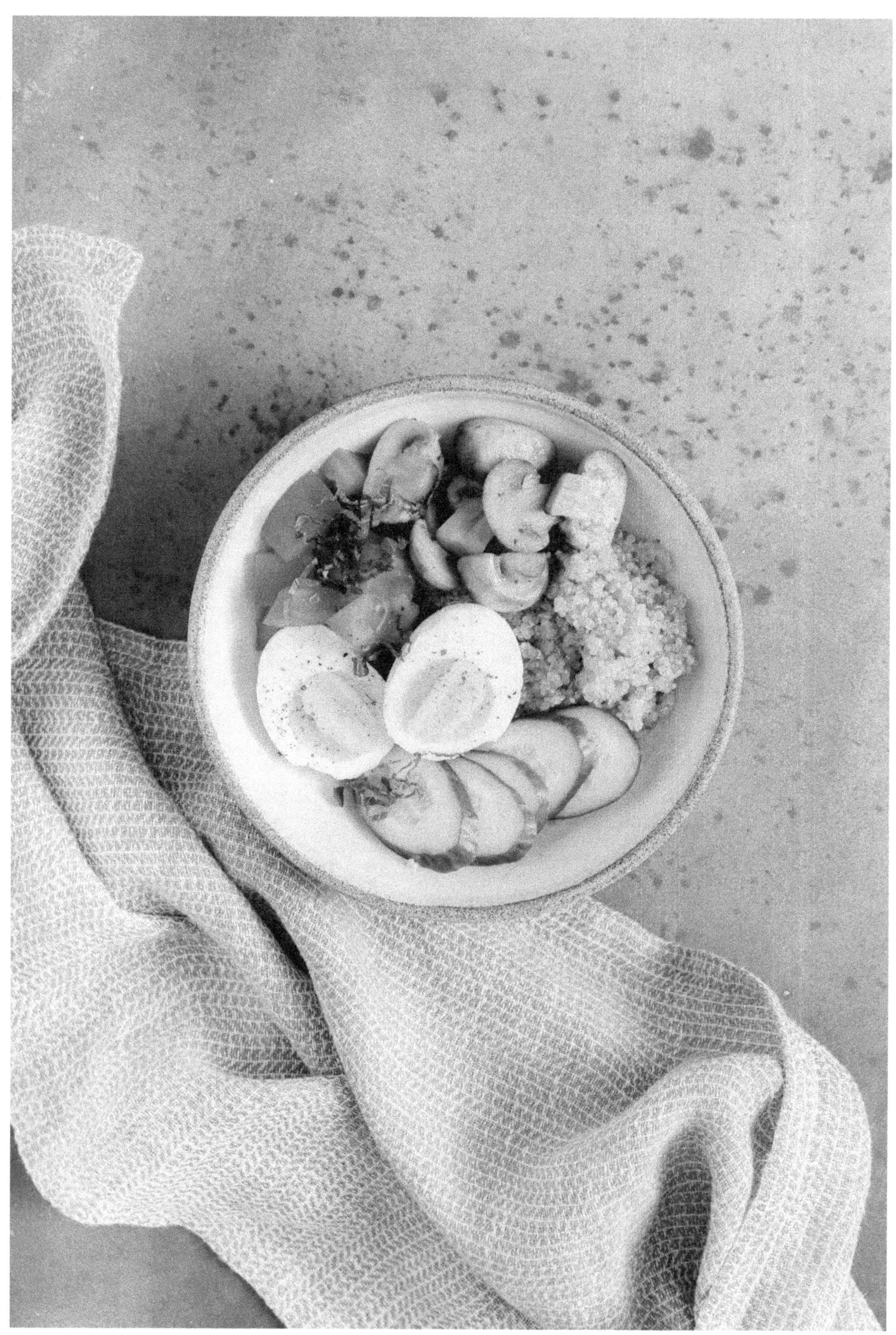

CHAPTER 1

Understanding Osteoporosis:

What is Osteoporosis?

Welcome to the enlightening journey of understanding osteoporosis—an ailment that silently threatens the strength and integrity of our skeletal system. As an orthopedist with years of experience, I am committed to unraveling the complexities of this condition, empowering you with knowledge that is not only enlightening but also transformative in safeguarding your bone health.

Osteoporosis, a term derived from Greek roots meaning "porous bones," encapsulates a condition characterized by the gradual weakening of bone density and structure.

While often perceived as an affliction of the elderly, osteoporosis transcends age, gender, and socioeconomic status, affecting millions worldwide.

At its core, osteoporosis undermines the very foundation of our skeletal system—a complex network of bones that provide structure, support, and mobility to our bodies. Imagine, if you will, a magnificent castle fortified by sturdy walls and battlements. Now, envision those walls gradually eroding, weakened by unseen forces—a poignant analogy for the insidious nature of osteoporosis.

But what exactly precipitates this gradual erosion of bone density? Allow me to shed light on the underlying mechanisms at play.

Our bones are dynamic entities, constantly undergoing a process of remodeling—where old bone tissue is resorbed and replaced by new bone. However, in individuals with osteoporosis, this delicate balance is disrupted, leading to an accelerated rate of bone resorption and a diminished capacity for bone formation.

The consequences of this imbalance are profound. Bones become porous and fragile, susceptible to fractures even from minimal trauma—a reality that poses significant implications for mobility, independence, and overall quality of life. From the debilitating fractures of the spine and hip to the subtle curvature of the spine known as kyphosis, the manifestations of osteoporosis are as varied as they are devastating.

Yet, amidst the shadows of despair, there exists a beacon of hope—a glimmer of possibility for prevention, intervention, and management. Through a comprehensive understanding of osteoporosis and its risk factors, we can empower ourselves to mitigate its impact and fortify our bones against its insidious onslaught.

How Osteoporosis Affects Seniors:

As individuals age, the risk of developing osteoporosis, a condition characterized by decreased bone density and increased bone fragility, becomes more pronounced. Osteoporosis affects seniors in several significant ways, each with profound implications for their health, mobility, and overall quality of life.

1. Increased Risk of Fractures:

Seniors with osteoporosis are at heightened risk of experiencing fractures, particularly in weight-bearing bones such as the hips, spine, and wrists. These fractures can occur even with minor falls or trauma and can have serious consequences, including prolonged pain, decreased mobility, and loss of independence. Hip fractures, in particular, are associated with a higher risk of mortality and can lead to significant disability and reduced quality of life.

2. Impaired Mobility and Function:

Osteoporosis-related fractures can severely impact seniors' mobility and functional independence. Fractures of the spine (vertebral compression fractures) can lead to a loss of height, stooped posture (kyphosis), and chronic back pain, making it challenging to perform daily activities such as walking, bending, and lifting. Fractures of the hip or pelvis can result in limited mobility, difficulty with weight-bearing activities, and an increased reliance on assistive devices such as canes or walkers.

3. Decreased Quality of Life:

Living with osteoporosis can significantly diminish seniors' overall quality of life. Chronic pain, functional limitations, and fear of falling can contribute to social isolation, depression, and anxiety. Seniors may experience a loss of independence and a reduced ability to engage in activities they once enjoyed, leading to feelings of frustration, helplessness, and decreased self-esteem.

4. Increased Healthcare Utilization and Costs:

Osteoporosis-related fractures impose a substantial burden on the healthcare system, resulting in increased hospitalizations, surgical interventions, and rehabilitation services for seniors. The management of osteoporosis requires ongoing medical monitoring, diagnostic testing (such as bone density scans), and pharmacological interventions (such as osteoporosis medications), all of which contribute to healthcare costs and resource utilization.

5. Higher Mortality Rates:

Osteoporosis is associated with higher mortality rates, particularly following hip fractures. Seniors who experience hip fractures have an increased risk of complications such as pneumonia, blood clots, and infections, which can contribute to premature death. Furthermore, the physical and psychological toll of osteoporosis-related fractures can exacerbate existing health conditions and decrease overall life expectancy.

In summary, osteoporosis significantly impacts seniors by increasing their risk of fractures, impairing mobility and function, diminishing quality of life, increasing healthcare utilization and costs, and contributing to higher mortality rates. Recognizing the multifaceted effects of osteoporosis on seniors is crucial for implementing effective prevention, screening, and management strategies to mitigate its impact and promote healthy aging.

Osteoporosis is a multifactorial condition influenced by a combination of genetic, lifestyle, and medical factors. Understanding these risk factors is essential for identifying individuals who may be at increased risk of developing osteoporosis and implementing preventive measures to maintain bone health. Below are the key risk factors associated with osteoporosis:

1. Age:

Age is one of the primary risk factors for osteoporosis. As individuals age, bone density naturally decreases, and bone remodeling processes become less efficient. Postmenopausal women and men over the age of 65 are at particularly high risk due to hormonal changes and age-related bone loss.

2. Gender:

Women are at higher risk of developing osteoporosis compared to men, primarily due to lower peak bone mass and hormonal changes associated with menopause. Estrogen plays a crucial role in maintaining bone density, and the decline in estrogen levels during menopause accelerates bone loss in women.

3. Family History and Genetics:

A family history of osteoporosis or fragility fractures can significantly increase an individual's risk of developing the condition. Genetic factors influence bone density, bone structure, and susceptibility to fractures, highlighting the importance of understanding familial predispositions to osteoporosis.

4. Hormonal Factors:

Hormonal imbalances or deficiencies can contribute to osteoporosis. In addition to estrogen deficiency in postmenopausal women, conditions such as hypogonadism (low testosterone levels in men), hyperthyroidism (excessive thyroid hormone production), and hyperparathyroidism (excessive parathyroid hormone production) can negatively impact bone health.

5. Nutritional Deficiencies:

Inadequate intake of calcium and vitamin D, essential nutrients for bone formation and maintenance, can increase the risk of osteoporosis. Chronic deficiencies in these nutrients can compromise bone mineralization and weaken bone structure, predisposing individuals to fractures and bone-related complications.

6. Lifestyle Factors:

Certain lifestyle choices and habits can contribute to the development of osteoporosis. These include smoking, excessive alcohol consumption, sedentary behavior, and low levels of physical activity. Smoking interferes with bone remodeling and reduces bone density, while excessive alcohol intake can impair calcium absorption and increase the risk of falls and fractures.

7. Medical Conditions and Medications:

Certain medical conditions and medications are associated with an increased risk of osteoporosis. These include rheumatoid arthritis, inflammatory bowel disease, celiac disease, chronic kidney disease, and endocrine disorders. Additionally, long-term use of glucocorticoid medications (such as prednisone) and certain anticonvulsant medications can have detrimental effects on bone health.

8. Body Composition:

Low body weight, a low body mass index (BMI), and a small frame size are risk factors for osteoporosis. Individuals with these characteristics may have less bone mass to begin with, making them more susceptible to bone loss and fractures as they age.

By recognizing and addressing these risk factors, individuals and healthcare professionals can take proactive steps to prevent osteoporosis, screen for early signs of bone loss, and implement strategies to maintain bone health throughout life. This comprehensive approach encompasses lifestyle modifications, nutritional interventions, medical management, and regular bone density screenings to reduce the burden of osteoporosis and promote healthy aging.

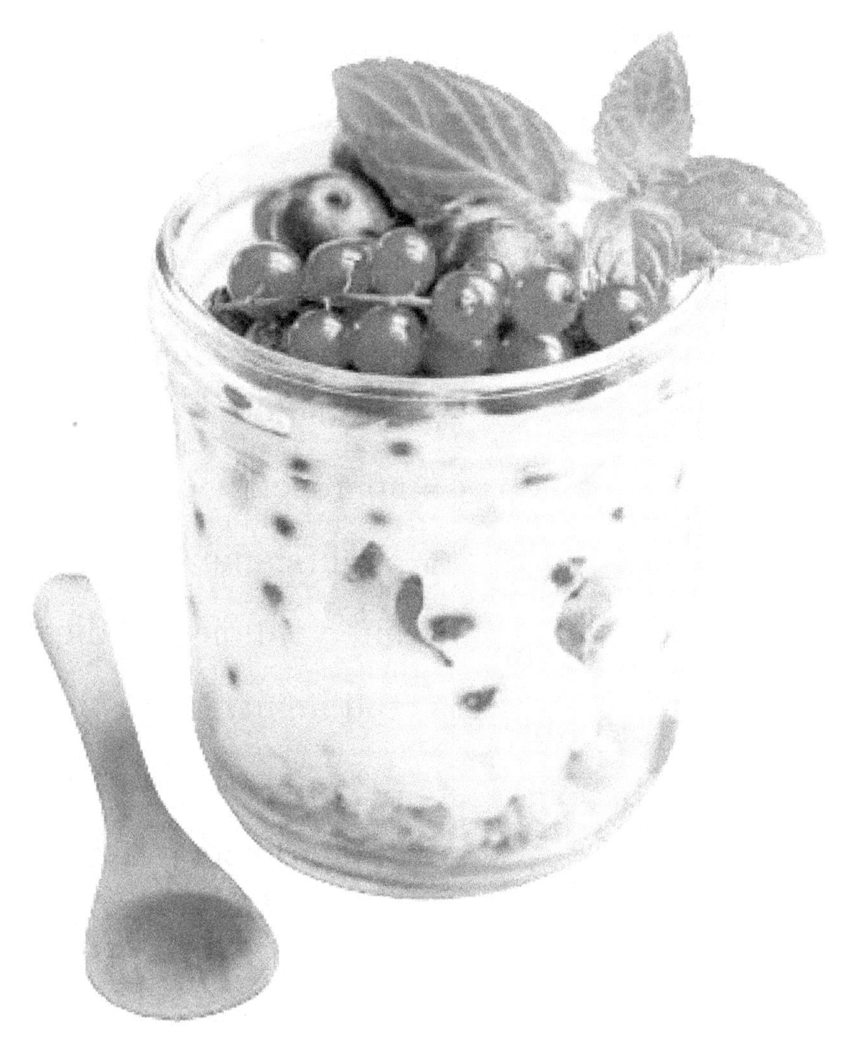

CHAPTER 2

The Role of Nutrition in Bone Health:

Let's delve into the crucial role that nutrition plays in maintaining optimal bone health.

Nutrition plays a fundamental role in supporting bone health throughout life, from childhood to old age. Bones are dynamic tissues that require a variety of nutrients to develop, grow, and maintain their strength and density. Adequate intake of key nutrients is essential for promoting bone formation, mineralization, and remodeling processes. Below are the key nutrients and dietary factors that contribute to bone health:

1. Calcium: Calcium is the primary mineral component of bones, accounting for approximately 99% of total body calcium. Adequate calcium intake is essential for building and maintaining strong bones and teeth. Dairy products such as milk, yogurt, and cheese are rich sources of calcium, but it can also be obtained from fortified plant-based alternatives, leafy green vegetables (such as kale and broccoli), tofu, almonds, and canned fish with bones (such as salmon and sardines).

2. Vitamin D:

Vitamin D plays a crucial role in calcium absorption and utilization, facilitating the incorporation of calcium into bone tissue. Sunlight exposure triggers vitamin D synthesis in the skin, but it can also be obtained from dietary sources such as fatty fish (e.g., salmon, mackerel), egg yolks, fortified dairy products, and fortified cereals. Adequate vitamin D levels are essential for maintaining bone density and reducing the risk of fractures.

3. Protein:

Protein is a key structural component of bones, providing the framework for bone formation and repair. Adequate protein intake is necessary for maintaining bone mass and supporting bone health. Good sources of protein include lean meats, poultry, fish, eggs, dairy products, legumes, nuts, and seeds. Balancing protein intake with calcium and other nutrients is important for optimizing bone health.

4. **Magnesium:** Magnesium is involved in bone mineralization and plays a role in regulating calcium metabolism. Consuming magnesium-rich foods such as leafy green vegetables, nuts, seeds, whole grains, and legumes can support bone health and help prevent osteoporosis.

5. Vitamin K:

Vitamin K is essential for synthesizing proteins involved in bone mineralization and reducing calcium loss from bones. Green leafy vegetables (such as kale, spinach, and collard greens), broccoli, Brussels sprouts, and fermented foods (such as natto) are rich dietary sources of vitamin K.

6. Phosphorus:

Phosphorus is another mineral that contributes to bone structure and strength.

It works in conjunction with calcium to form hydroxyapatite crystals, the mineral matrix of bone tissue. Phosphorus is abundant in protein-rich foods such as meat, poultry, fish, dairy products, nuts, seeds, and whole grains.

7. Micronutrients and Phytonutrients:

In addition to the macronutrients mentioned above, several micronutrients and phytonutrients play roles in bone health. These include vitamin C (found in citrus fruits, strawberries, bell peppers), vitamin A (found in sweet potatoes, carrots, spinach), zinc (found in meat, seafood, nuts, seeds), and antioxidants (found in colorful fruits and vegetables).

In summary, nutrition plays a critical role in supporting bone health by providing the essential nutrients needed for bone formation, mineralization, and maintenance. A well-balanced diet rich in calcium, vitamin D, protein, magnesium, vitamin K, phosphorus, and other micronutrients is key to promoting optimal bone health and reducing the risk of osteoporosis and fractures throughout life. Incorporating a variety of nutrient-dense foods into your diet and maintaining a healthy lifestyle are essential strategies for supporting strong and resilient bones.

While certain foods are beneficial for bone health, there are also foods that should be limited or avoided to promote optimal bone health. Here are some foods to avoid or consume in moderation:

1. High-Sodium Foods:

Consuming high-sodium foods can increase urinary calcium excretion and promote calcium loss from bones, potentially weakening bone density over time. Processed foods such as canned soups, processed meats, snack foods, and fast food meals are often high in sodium. Limiting the intake of these foods can help prevent excessive calcium loss and preserve bone health.

2. Carbonated Beverages:

Carbonated beverages, particularly those sweetened with sugar or high-fructose corn syrup, have been associated with decreased bone mineral density and increased risk of fractures. The phosphoric acid found in many carbonated drinks may interfere with calcium absorption and contribute to bone demineralization. Opt for water, herbal teas, or calcium-fortified beverages as healthier alternatives.

3. Excessive Alcohol:

Chronic alcohol consumption can adversely affect bone health by interfering with calcium metabolism, reducing bone formation, and increasing the risk of falls and fractures. Heavy alcohol intake can also impair liver function, leading to vitamin D deficiency and secondary osteoporosis. Limit alcohol consumption to moderate levels (no more than one drink per day for women and two drinks per day for men) to minimize its negative impact on bone health.

4. Caffeine:

While moderate caffeine intake is generally considered safe, excessive consumption of caffeinated beverages (such as coffee, tea, and energy drinks) may interfere with calcium absorption and increase urinary calcium excretion. Aim to limit caffeine intake to no more than 300 milligrams per day (equivalent to about two to three cups of coffee) and balance it with calcium-rich foods to mitigate its potential effects on bone health.

5. High-Protein Diets:

While protein is important for bone health, consuming excessively high amounts of protein, especially animal-based protein, may increase urinary calcium excretion and potentially weaken bones over time. Instead of relying solely on animal protein sources, incorporate a variety of protein-rich foods into your diet, including plant-based sources such as legumes, nuts, seeds, and tofu.

6. Foods High in Oxalates:

Some foods contain high levels of oxalates, compounds that can bind to calcium and inhibit its absorption in the body. Examples of foods high in oxalates include spinach, rhubarb, beet greens, and Swiss chard. While these foods offer other nutritional benefits, consuming them in excess may interfere with calcium absorption and negatively impact bone health. Enjoy these foods in moderation as part of a balanced diet.

7. Excessive Vitamin A:

While vitamin A is important for overall health, consuming excessive amounts of preformed vitamin A (retinol) from animal-based foods or supplements may have adverse effects on bone health and increase the risk of fractures.

Limit intake of liver and organ meats, which are particularly high in vitamin A, and focus on obtaining vitamin A from beta-carotene-rich fruits and vegetables such as carrots, sweet potatoes, and dark leafy greens.

By being mindful of these foods and making informed dietary choices, you can support optimal bone health and reduce the risk of osteoporosis and fractures in the long term. A balanced diet rich in calcium, vitamin D, protein, magnesium, vitamin K, and other essential nutrients, along with regular physical activity and a healthy lifestyle, is key to maintaining strong and resilient bones throughout life. If you have specific concerns about your diet or bone health, consult with a healthcare professional or registered dietitian for personalized guidance and recommendations.

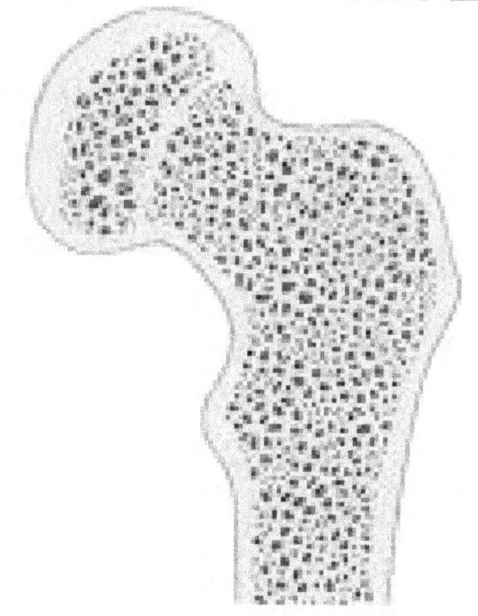

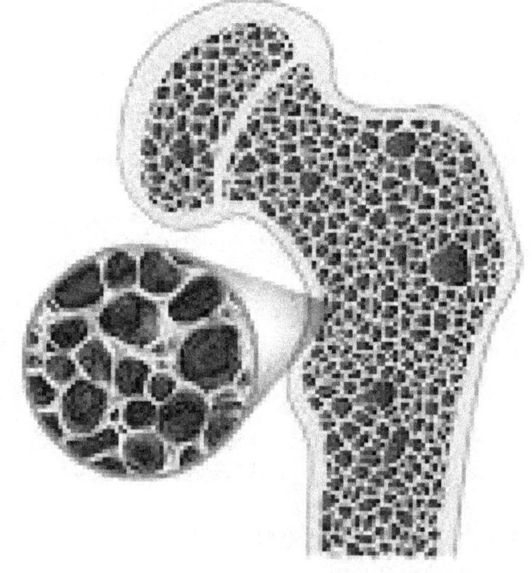

Smoothie and juice recipes:

Green Goddess Smoothie:

Ingredients:

- 1 cup spinach
- 1/2 cup kale
- 1/2 ripe avocado
- 1/2 cup cucumber, chopped
- 1/2 cup unsweetened almond milk
- 1/4 teaspoon ground cinnamon
- 1 tablespoon chia seeds

Preparation:

1) Combine all ingredients in a blender and blend until smooth.
2) Add more almond milk if needed for desired consistency.

Number of servings: 1

Nutritional value per serving:

- Calories: 150
- Protein: 5g
- Fat: 10g
- Carbohydrates: 12g
- Fiber: 8g

Preparation time: 5 minutes

Berry Blast Smoothie:

Ingredients:

- 1/2 cup mixed berries (such as strawberries, blueberries, raspberries)
- 1/2 banana
- 1/2 cup plain Greek yogurt (low-fat)
- 1/2 cup unsweetened almond milk
- 1 tablespoon flaxseeds
- 1 teaspoon honey (optional)

1) Combine all ingredients in a blender and blend until smooth.
2) Add more almond milk if needed for desired consistency.

Number of servings: 1

Nutritional value per serving:

- Calories: 180
- Protein: 10g
- Fat: 5g
- Carbohydrates: 25g
- Fiber: 6g

Preparation time: 5 minutes

Tropical Sunshine Smoothie:

Ingredients:

- 1/2 cup pineapple chunks
- 1/2 ripe mango, diced
- 1/2 cup coconut water
- 1/2 cup plain Greek yogurt (low-fat)
- 1 tablespoon shredded coconut (unsweetened)
- 1/4 teaspoon turmeric powder

Preparation:

1) Combine all ingredients in a blender and blend until smooth.
2) Add ice cubes if desired for a colder texture.

Number of servings: 1

Nutritional value per serving:

- Calories: 160
- Protein: 8g
- Fat: 4g
- Carbohydrates: 25g
- Fiber: 5g

Preparation time: 5 minutes

Protein Power Smoothie

Ingredients:

- ➢ 1/2 cup cooked quinoa
- ➢ 1/2 cup unsweetened almond milk
- ➢ 1/2 banana
- ➢ 1 tablespoon almond butter
- ➢ 1 teaspoon honey (optional)
- ➢ 1/4 teaspoon vanilla extract

Preparation:

1) Combine all ingredients in a blender and blend until smooth.
2) Add more almond milk if needed for desired consistency.

Number of servings: 1

Nutritional value per serving:

- Calories: 250
- Protein: 12g
- Fat: 8g
- Carbohydrates: 35g
- Fiber: 5g

Preparation time: 5 minutes

Citrus Sunrise Juice

Ingredients:

- ➢ 1 orange, peeled and segmented
- ➢ 1/2 grapefruit, peeled and segmented
- ➢ 1/2 lemon, peeled
- ➢ 1/2 inch fresh ginger root
- ➢ 1/2 cup water

Preparation:

1) Combine all ingredients in a juicer and process until smooth.
2) Strain the juice to remove any pulp if desired.

Number of servings: 1

Nutritional value per serving:

- Calories: 80
- Protein: 2g
- Fat: 1g
- Carbohydrates: 20g
- Fiber: 5g

Preparation time: 5 minutes

Creamy Almond Joy Smoothie

Ingredients:

- 1/2 cup unsweetened almond milk
- 1/2 ripe banana
- 1 tablespoon almond butter
- 1 tablespoon cocoa powder (unsweetened)
- 1 tablespoon shredded coconut (unsweetened)
- 1 teaspoon honey (optional)

Preparation:

1) Combine all ingredients in a blender and blend until smooth.

2) Add ice cubes if desired for a colder texture.

Number of servings: 1

Nutritional value per serving:

- Calories: 200
- Protein: 6g
- Fat: 12g
- Carbohydrates: 20g
- Fiber: 6g

Preparation time: 5 minutes

Peachy Green Smoothie

Ingredients:

- 1/2 cup frozen peaches
- 1/2 cup spinach
- 1/2 cup plain Greek yogurt (low-fat)
- 1/2 cup unsweetened almond milk
- 1 tablespoon hemp seeds
- 1 teaspoon honey (optional)

Preparation:

1) Combine all ingredients in a blender and blend until smooth.

2) Add more almond milk if needed for desired consistency.

Number of servings: 1

Nutritional value per serving:

- Calories: 180
- Protein: 10g
- Fat: 5g
- Carbohydrates: 25g
- Fiber: 6g

Preparation time: 5 minutes

Golden Glow Turmeric Smoothie

Ingredients:

- 1/2 cup mango chunks
- 1/2 banana
- 1/2 teaspoon ground turmeric
- 1/2 teaspoon ground cinnamon
- 1/2 cup plain Greek yogurt (low-fat)
- 1/2 cup unsweetened almond milk
- 1 teaspoon honey (optional)

Preparation:

1) Combine all ingredients in a blender and blend until smooth.

2) Adjust sweetness with honey if desired.

Number of servings: 1

Nutritional value per serving:

- Calories: 170
- Protein: 8g
- Fat: 4g
- Carbohydrates: 25g
- Fiber: 5g

Preparation time: 5 minutes

Ingredients:

- 1/2 cup beetroot, peeled and chopped
- 1/2 cup mixed berries (such as strawberries, blueberries, raspberries)
- 1/2 inch fresh ginger root
- 1/2 cup water

Preparation:

1) Combine all ingredients in a juicer and process until smooth.
2) Strain the juice to remove any pulp if desired.

Number of servings: 1

Nutritional value per serving:

- Calories: 90
- Protein: 2g
- Fat: 1g
- Carbohydrates: 20g
- Fiber: 5g

Preparation time: 5 minutes

Creamy Berry Almond Juice

Ingredients:

- 1/2 cup mixed berries (such as strawberries, blueberries, raspberries)
- 1/2 ripe banana
- 1/2 cup unsweetened almond milk
- 1 tablespoon almond butter
- 1/4 teaspoon vanilla extract

Preparation:

1) Combine all ingredients in a blender and blend until smooth.
2) Add more almond milk if needed for desired consistency.

Number of servings: 1

Nutritional value per serving:

- Calories: 200
- Protein: 6g
- Fat: 12g
- Carbohydrates: 20g
- Fiber: 6g

Preparation time: 5 minutes

These nutrient-rich smoothie and juice recipes are not only delicious but also packed with essential vitamins, minerals, and antioxidants to support bone health and overall well-being. Enjoy them as part of a balanced diet to nourish your body and promote optimal health.

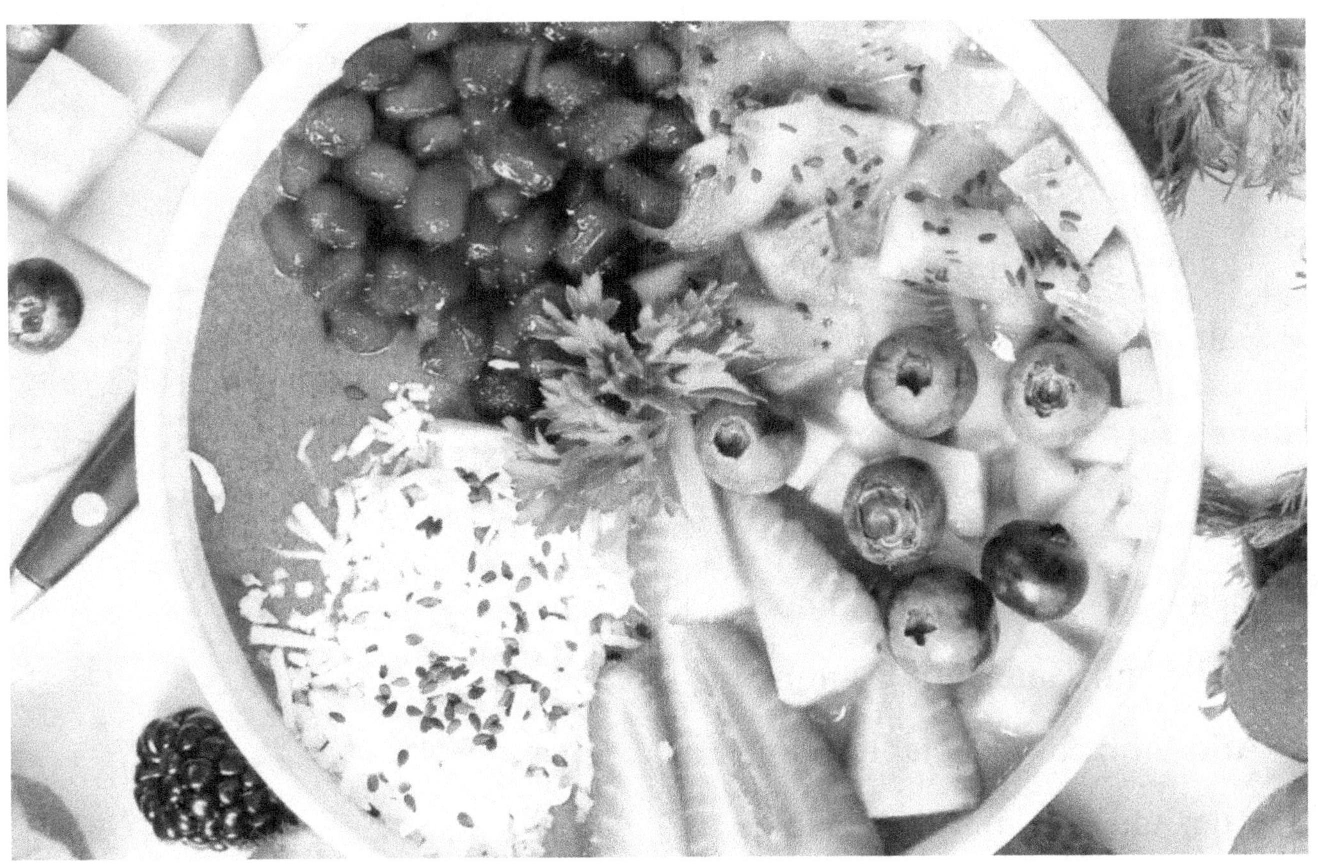

Quinoa and Vegetable Soup:

Ingredients:

- 1 cup cooked quinoa
- 2 cups low-sodium vegetable broth
- 1 cup mixed vegetables (carrots, celery, bell peppers)
- 1/2 cup kale, chopped
- 1 teaspoon olive oil
- 1 clove garlic, minced
- Salt and pepper to taste

Preparation:

1) In a pot, heat olive oil over medium heat. Add minced garlic and sauté until fragrant.
2) Add mixed vegetables and kale, and sauté until vegetables are tender.
3) Add cooked quinoa and vegetable broth to the pot. Bring to a simmer and cook for 10-15 minutes.
4) Season with salt and pepper to taste.

Number of servings: 4

Nutritional value per serving:

- Calories: 120
- Protein: 4g
- Fat: 3g
- Carbohydrates: 20g
- Fiber: 5g

Cooking time: 20 minutes

Ingredients:

- ➢ 2 cups mixed greens (spinach, arugula, kale)
- ➢ 1/2 cup firm tofu, cubed
- ➢ 1 tablespoon miso paste
- ➢ 1 tablespoon rice vinegar
- ➢ 1 teaspoon sesame oil
- ➢ 1 tablespoon sesame seeds

Preparation:

1) In a small bowl, whisk together miso paste, rice vinegar, and sesame oil to make the dressing.
2) Toss mixed greens and cubed tofu in the dressing until evenly coated.
3) Sprinkle sesame seeds on top and serve.

Number of servings: 2

Nutritional value per serving:

- Calories: 120
- Protein: 8g
- Fat: 7g
- Carbohydrates: 10g
- Fiber: 4g

Cooking time: 10 minutes

Roasted Butternut Squash Soup

Ingredients:

- ➢ 1 small butternut squash, peeled and cubed
- ➢ 1 onion, diced
- ➢ 2 cloves garlic, minced
- ➢ 4 cups low-sodium vegetable broth
- ➢ 1 tablespoon olive oil
- ➢ 1/2 teaspoon ground cinnamon
- ➢ Salt and pepper to taste

Preparation:

1) Preheat oven to 400°F (200°C). Place cubed butternut squash on a baking sheet and

drizzle with olive oil. Season with salt, pepper, and ground cinnamon.

2) Roast squash in the oven for 25-30 minutes, or until tender and caramelized.

3) In a pot, heat olive oil over medium heat. Add diced onion and minced garlic, and sauté until translucent.

4) Add roasted butternut squash and vegetable broth to the pot. Bring to a simmer and cook for 10-15 minutes.

5) Use an immersion blender to puree the soup until smooth. Season with salt and pepper to taste.

Number of servings: 4

Nutritional value per serving:

- Calories: 150
- Protein: 3g
- Fat: 4g
- Carbohydrates: 30g
- Fiber: 5g

Cooking time: 45 minutes

Spinach and Strawberry Salad

Ingredients:

- 2 cups baby spinach
- 1 cup strawberries, sliced
- 1/4 cup walnuts, chopped
- 1/4 cup feta cheese, crumbled
- 1 tablespoon balsamic vinegar
- 1 tablespoon olive oil

Preparation:

1) In a large bowl, combine baby spinach, sliced strawberries, chopped walnuts, and crumbled feta cheese.

2) Drizzle balsamic vinegar and olive oil over the salad and toss until evenly coated.

3) Serve immediately.

Number of servings: 2

Nutritional value per serving:

- Calories: 160
- Protein: 5g
- Fat: 10g
- Carbohydrates: 15g
- Fiber: 5g

Cooking time: 10 minutes

Broccoli and White Bean Soup

Ingredients:

- ➢ 2 cups broccoli florets
- ➢ 1 can white beans, drained and rinsed
- ➢ 1 onion, diced
- ➢ 2 cloves garlic, minced
- ➢ 4 cups low-sodium vegetable broth
- ➢ 1 tablespoon olive oil
- ➢ Salt and pepper to taste

Preparation:

1) In a pot, heat olive oil over medium heat. Add diced onion and minced garlic, and sauté until translucent.
2) Add broccoli florets and white beans to the pot. Cook for 5-7 minutes, stirring occasionally.
3) Add vegetable broth to the pot and bring to a simmer. Cook for an additional 10-15 minutes, or until broccoli is tender.
4) Use an immersion blender to puree the soup until smooth. Season with salt and pepper to taste.

Number of servings: 4

Nutritional value per serving:

- Calories: 130
- Protein: 7g
- Fat: 3g
- Carbohydrates: 20g
- Fiber: 6g

Cooking time: 30 minutes

Ingredients:

- 2 cups cooked chickpeas
- 1 cucumber, diced
- 1 tomato, diced
- 1/4 cup red onion, thinly sliced
- 1/4 cup Kalamata olives, pitted
- 1/4 cup feta cheese, crumbled
- 2 tablespoons lemon juice
- 1 tablespoon olive oil
- 1 teaspoon dried oregano
- Salt and pepper to taste

Preparation:

1) In a large bowl, combine cooked chickpeas, diced cucumber, diced tomato, thinly sliced red onion, pitted Kalamata olives, and crumbled feta cheese.

2) Drizzle lemon juice and olive oil over the salad. Sprinkle dried oregano, salt, and pepper to taste.

3) Toss until all ingredients are evenly coated.

4) Serve chilled or at room temperature.

Number of servings: 4

Nutritional value per serving:

- Calories: 200
- Protein: 9g
- Fat: 7g
- Carbohydrates: 25g
- Fiber: 7g

Cooking time: 15 minutes

Ingredients:

- 4 large tomatoes, diced
- 1 onion, diced
- 2 cloves garlic, minced
- 4 cups low-sodium vegetable broth
- 1/4 cup fresh basil leaves, chopped
- 2 tablespoons olive oil
- Salt and pepper to taste

Preparation:

1) In a pot, heat olive oil over medium heat. Add diced onion and minced garlic, and sauté until translucent.
2) Add diced tomatoes to the pot and cook for 5-7 minutes, until softened.
3) Add vegetable broth to the pot and bring to a simmer. Cook for an additional 10-15 minutes.
4) Use an immersion blender to puree the soup until smooth. Stir in chopped basil leaves and season with salt and pepper to taste.

Number of servings: 4

Nutritional value per serving:

- Calories: 100
- Protein: 3g
- Fat: 5g
- Carbohydrates: 15g
- Fiber: 5g

Cooking time: 30 minutes

Ingredients:

- ➤ 1 cup cooked quinoa
- ➤ 1/2 cup cherry tomatoes, halved
- ➤ 1/2 cup cucumber, diced
- ➤ 1/2 cup bell peppers (red, yellow, or orange), diced
- ➤ 1/4 cup red cabbage, shredded
- ➤ 1/4 cup carrots, shredded
- ➤ 2 tablespoons lemon juice
- ➤ 1 tablespoon olive oil
- ➤ 1 tablespoon fresh parsley, chopped
- ➤ Salt and pepper to taste

Preparation:

1) In a large bowl, combine cooked quinoa, cherry tomatoes, diced cucumber, diced bell peppers, shredded red cabbage, and shredded carrots.

2) In a small bowl, whisk together lemon juice, olive oil, chopped parsley, salt, and pepper to make the dressing.

3) Drizzle the dressing over the salad and toss until all ingredients are evenly coated.

4) Serve chilled or at room temperature.

Number of servings: 4

Nutritional value per serving:

- Calories: 150
- Protein: 5g
- Fat: 5g
- Carbohydrates: 20g
- Fiber: 5g

Cooking time: 20 minutes

Ingredients:

- ➤ 1 head cauliflower, chopped
- ➤ 1 onion, diced
- ➤ 2 cloves garlic, minced
- ➤ 4 cups low-sodium vegetable broth
- ➤ 1/2 cup unsweetened almond milk
- ➤ 2 tablespoons nutritional yeast
- ➤ 1 tablespoon olive oil
- ➤ Salt and pepper to taste

Preparation:

1) In a pot, heat olive oil over medium heat. Add diced onion and minced garlic, and sauté until translucent.
2) Add chopped cauliflower to the pot and cook for 5-7 minutes, until slightly softened.
3) Add vegetable broth to the pot and bring to a simmer. Cook for an additional 10-15 minutes, or until cauliflower is tender.
4) Use an immersion blender to puree the soup until smooth. Stir in unsweetened almond milk and nutritional yeast. Season with salt and pepper to taste.

Number of servings: 4

Nutritional value per serving:

- Calories: 100
- Protein: 5g
- Fat: 4g
- Carbohydrates: 15g
- Fiber: 5g

Cooking time: 30 minutes

Ingredients:

- 1 can chickpeas, drained and rinsed
- 1 avocado, diced
- 1/2 cup cherry tomatoes, halved
- 1/4 cup red onion, diced
- 2 tablespoons lemon juice
- 1 tablespoon olive oil
- 1 tablespoon fresh cilantro, chopped
- Salt and pepper to taste

Preparation:

1) In a large bowl, combine drained chickpeas, diced avocado, halved cherry tomatoes, and diced red onion.
2) In a small bowl, whisk together lemon juice, olive oil, chopped cilantro, salt, and pepper to make the dressing.
3) Drizzle the dressing over the salad and toss until all ingredients are evenly coated.
4) Serve chilled or at room temperature.

Number of servings: 4

Nutritional value per serving:

- Calories: 180
- Protein: 7g
- Fat: 8g
- Carbohydrates: 20g
- Fiber: 7g

Cooking time: 15 minutes

Ingredients:

- ➤ 1 cup dried lentils
- ➤ 2 carrots, diced
- ➤ 2 celery stalks, diced
- ➤ 1 onion, diced
- ➤ 2 cloves garlic, minced
- ➤ 4 cups low-sodium vegetable broth
- ➤ 1 teaspoon olive oil
- ➤ 1 teaspoon ground cumin
- ➤ Salt and pepper to taste

Preparation:

1) In a pot, heat olive oil over medium heat. Add diced onion and minced garlic, and sauté until translucent.
2) Add diced carrots and celery to the pot, and cook for 5 minutes, stirring occasionally.
3) Rinse lentils under cold water and add them to the pot. Stir in ground cumin.
4) Add vegetable broth to the pot and bring to a boil. Reduce heat and simmer for 20-25 minutes, or until lentils are tender.
5) Season with salt and pepper to taste.

Number of servings: 4

Nutritional value per serving:

- Calories: 200
- Protein: 10g
- Fat: 2g
- Carbohydrates: 35g
- Fiber: 12g

Cooking time: 35 minutes

Ingredients:

- 4 cups arugula
- 1 pear, thinly sliced
- 1/4 cup walnuts, chopped
- 1/4 cup dried cranberries
- 2 tablespoons balsamic vinegar
- 1 tablespoon olive oil
- Salt and pepper to taste

Preparation:

1) In a large bowl, combine arugula, thinly sliced pear, chopped walnuts, and dried cranberries.
2) In a small bowl, whisk together balsamic vinegar, olive oil, salt, and pepper to make the dressing.
3) Drizzle the dressing over the salad and toss until all ingredients are evenly coated.
4) Serve immediately.

Number of servings: 2

Nutritional value per serving:

- Calories: 180
- Protein: 4g
- Fat: 10g
- Carbohydrates: 25g
- Fiber: 6g

Cooking time: 10 minutes

Sweet Potato and Black Bean Soup

Ingredients:

- 2 sweet potatoes, peeled and diced
- 1 can black beans, drained and rinsed
- 1 onion, diced
- 2 cloves garlic, minced
- 4 cups low-sodium vegetable broth
- 1 tablespoon olive oil
- 1 teaspoon ground cumin

Preparation:

1) In a pot, heat olive oil over medium heat. Add diced onion and minced garlic, and sauté until translucent.
2) Add diced sweet potatoes to the pot, and cook for 5 minutes, stirring occasionally.
3) Rinse black beans under cold water and add them to the pot. Stir in ground cumin.
4) Add vegetable broth to the pot and bring to a boil. Reduce heat and simmer for 20-25 minutes, or until sweet potatoes are tender.
5) Season with salt and pepper to taste.

Number of servings: 4

Nutritional value per serving:

- Calories: 180
- Protein: 7g
- Fat: 3g
- Carbohydrates: 35g
- Fiber: 10g

Cooking time: 35 minutes

Cucumber and Quinoa Salad

Ingredients:

➤ 2 cups cooked quinoa
➤ 1 cucumber, diced
➤ 1/2 cup cherry tomatoes, halved
➤ 1/4 cup red onion, thinly sliced
➤ 2 tablespoons lemon juice
➤ 1 tablespoon olive oil
➤ 1 tablespoon fresh dill, chopped
➤ Salt and pepper to taste

Preparation:

1) In a large bowl, combine cooked quinoa, diced cucumber, halved cherry

tomatoes, and thinly sliced red onion.

2) In a small bowl, whisk together lemon juice, olive oil, chopped dill, salt, and pepper to make the dressing.

3) Drizzle the dressing over the salad and toss until all ingredients are evenly coated.

4) Serve chilled or at room temperature.

Number of servings: 4

Nutritional value per serving:

- Calories: 160
- Protein: 5g
- Fat: 6g
- Carbohydrates: 25g
- Fiber: 5g

Cooking time: 20 minutes

Creamy Tomato Basil Salad

Ingredients:

- ➢ 2 cups cherry tomatoes, halved
- ➢ 1/2 cup fresh mozzarella balls
- ➢ 1/4 cup fresh basil leaves, torn
- ➢ 2 tablespoons balsamic vinegar
- ➢ 1 tablespoon olive oil
- ➢ Salt and pepper to taste

Preparation:

1) In a large bowl, combine halved cherry tomatoes, fresh mozzarella balls, and torn basil leaves.

2) In a small bowl, whisk together balsamic vinegar, olive oil, salt, and pepper to make the dressing.

3) Drizzle the dressing over the salad and toss until all ingredients are evenly coated.

4) Serve immediately.

Nutritional value per serving:

- Calories: 180
- Protein: 8g
- Fat: 12g
- Carbohydrates: 15g
- Fiber: 4g

Cooking time: 10 minutes

These soups and salads are not only delicious but also packed with essential nutrients to support bone health and overall well-being. Enjoy them as part of a balanced diet to nourish your body and promote optimal health.

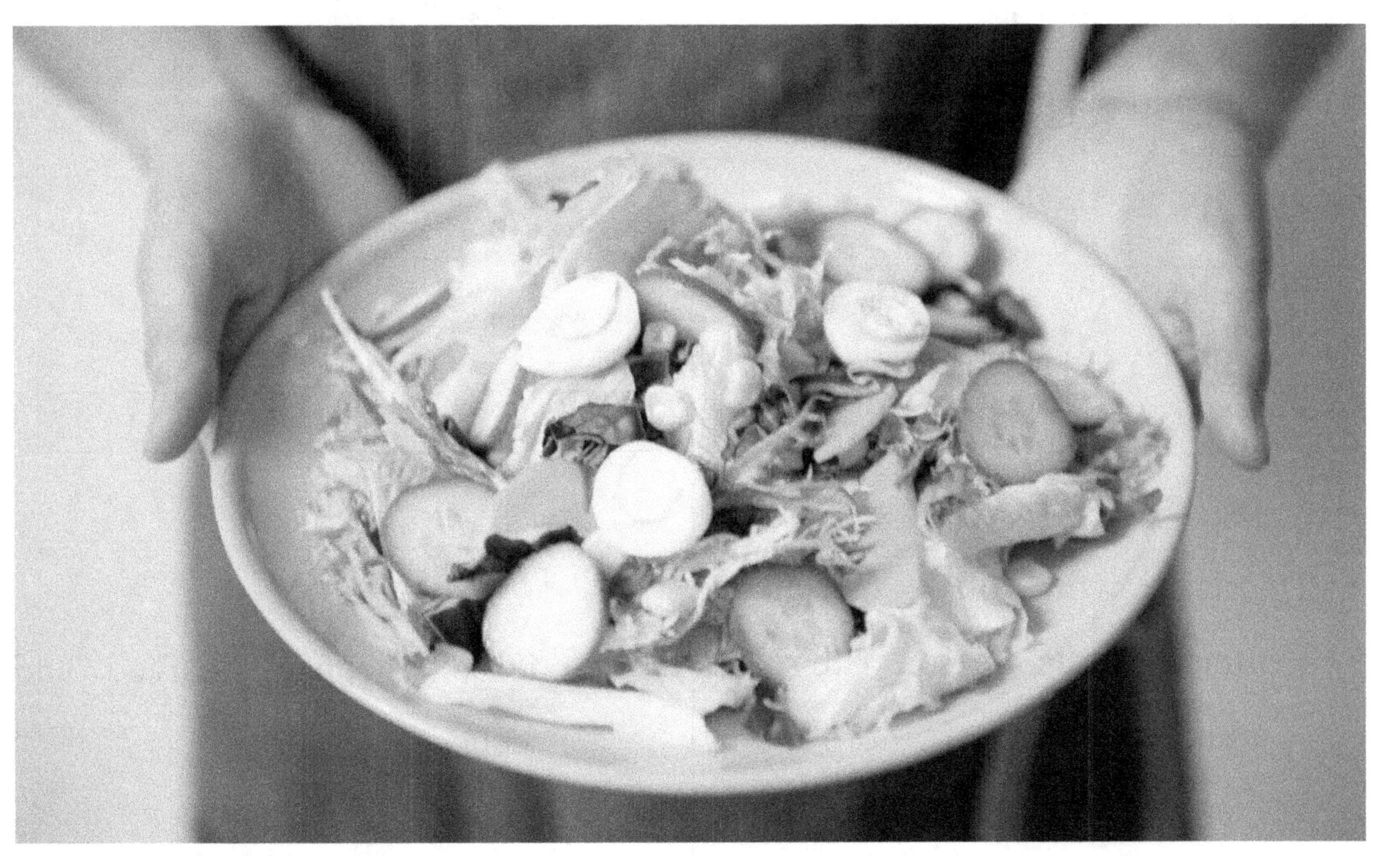

Salmon and Asparagus Bake

Ingredients:

- 4 salmon fillets
- 1 bunch asparagus, trimmed
- 2 tablespoons olive oil
- 2 cloves garlic, minced
- 1 lemon, sliced
- Salt and pepper to taste

Preparation:

1) Preheat the oven to 400°F (200°C). Place salmon fillets and asparagus on a baking sheet.
2) Drizzle with olive oil and minced garlic. Season with salt and pepper.
3) Place lemon slices on top of the salmon.
4) Bake for 15-20 minutes, or until salmon is cooked through and asparagus is tender.

Number of servings: 4

Nutritional value per serving:

- Calories: 250
- Protein: 25g
- Fat: 15g
- Carbohydrates: 5g
- Fiber: 2g

Cooking time: 20 minutes

Quinoa Stuffed Bell Peppers

Ingredients:

- 4 bell peppers, halved and seeded
- 1 cup cooked quinoa
- 1 can black beans, drained and rinsed

- ➢ 1 cup diced tomatoes
- ➢ 1/2 cup corn kernels
- ➢ 1/4 cup chopped cilantro
- ➢ 1 teaspoon cumin
- ➢ 1/2 teaspoon chili powder
- ➢ Salt and pepper to taste

1) Preheat the oven to 375°F (190°C). Place bell pepper halves in a baking dish.
2) In a bowl, mix cooked quinoa, black beans, diced tomatoes, corn kernels, chopped cilantro, cumin, chili powder, salt, and pepper.
3) Stuff each bell pepper half with the quinoa mixture.
4) Cover the baking dish with foil and bake for 30-35 minutes, or until bell peppers are tender.

Number of servings: 4

Nutritional value per serving:

- Calories: 280
- Protein: 10g
- Fat: 2g
- Carbohydrates: 55g
- Fiber: 10g

Cooking time: 40 minutes

Lemon Herb Chicken with Roasted Vegetables

Ingredients:

- ➢ 4 boneless, skinless chicken breasts
- ➢ 2 tablespoons olive oil
- ➢ 2 cloves garlic, minced
- ➢ 1 lemon, juiced and zested
- ➢ 1 tablespoon fresh thyme, chopped
- ➢ 1 tablespoon fresh rosemary, chopped
- ➢ 2 cups mixed vegetables (carrots, Brussels sprouts, potatoes)
- ➢ Salt and pepper to taste

1) Preheat the oven to 400°F (200°C). Place chicken breasts and mixed vegetables on a baking sheet.
2) In a small bowl, whisk together olive oil, minced garlic, lemon juice, lemon zest, chopped thyme, chopped rosemary, salt, and pepper.
3) Drizzle the lemon herb mixture over the chicken and vegetables.
4) Bake for 25-30 minutes, or until chicken is cooked through and vegetables are tender.

Number of servings: 4

Nutritional value per serving:

- Calories: 280
- Protein: 30g
- Fat: 10g
- Carbohydrates: 15g
- Fiber: 5g

Cooking time: 30 minutes

Vegetable Stir-Fry with Tofu

Ingredients:

- 1 block extra-firm tofu, pressed and cubed
- 2 tablespoons soy sauce
- 1 tablespoon sesame oil
- 2 cups mixed vegetables (broccoli, bell peppers, snap peas)
- 2 cloves garlic, minced
- 1 tablespoon ginger, minced
- 2 tablespoons hoisin sauce
- Cooked brown rice or quinoa for serving

Preparation:

1) In a bowl, toss cubed tofu with soy sauce and sesame oil. Let marinate for 15 minutes.
2) Heat a large skillet or wok over medium-high heat. Add marinated tofu and cook until

golden brown on all sides. Remove tofu from the skillet and set aside.

3) In the same skillet, add mixed vegetables, minced garlic, and minced ginger. Stir-fry until vegetables are tender-crisp.

4) Add cooked tofu back to the skillet and stir in hoisin sauce. Cook for an additional 2-3 minutes.

5) Serve stir-fry over cooked brown rice or quinoa.

Number of servings: 4

Nutritional value per serving:

- Calories: 300
- Protein: 20g
- Fat: 10g
- Carbohydrates: 35g
- Fiber: 8g

Cooking time: 25 minutes

Turkey and Vegetable Skewers

Ingredients:

- 1 lb turkey breast, cut into cubes
- 2 bell peppers, cut into chunks
- 1 red onion, cut into chunks
- 1 zucchini, sliced
- 8 cherry tomatoes
- 2 tablespoons olive oil
- 1 teaspoon paprika
- 1 teaspoon garlic powder
- Salt and pepper to taste

Preparation:

1) Preheat the grill or grill pan over medium-high heat.

2) In a bowl, toss turkey cubes and vegetables with olive oil, paprika, garlic powder, salt, and pepper.

3) Thread turkey cubes and vegetables onto skewers,

alternating between each ingredient.

4) Grill skewers for 10-12 minutes, turning occasionally, until turkey is cooked through and vegetables are tender.

- Calories: 220
- Protein: 30g
- Fat: 8g
- Carbohydrates: 10g
- Fiber: 3g

Eggplant Parmesan

Ingredients:

- 2 large eggplants, sliced
- 2 eggs, beaten
- 1 cup whole wheat breadcrumbs
- 1 cup marinara sauce
- 1 cup shredded mozzarella cheese
- 1/4 cup grated Parmesan cheese
- Fresh basil leaves for garnish
- Salt and pepper to taste

Preparation:

1) Preheat the oven to 375°F (190°C). Line a baking sheet with parchment paper.

2) Dip eggplant slices into beaten eggs, then coat with whole wheat breadcrumbs. Place on the prepared baking sheet.

3) Bake eggplant slices for 15-20 minutes, or until golden brown and tender.

4) In a baking dish, spread a layer of marinara sauce. Arrange baked eggplant slices on top.

5) Top eggplant slices with shredded mozzarella cheese and grated Parmesan cheese.

6) Bake for an additional 15 minutes, or until cheese is melted and bubbly.

7) Garnish with fresh basil leaves before serving.

Number of servings: 4

Nutritional value per serving:

- Calories: 280
- Protein: 15g
- Fat: 10g
- Carbohydrates: 35g
- Fiber: 8g

Cooking time: 40 minutes

Spinach and Feta Stuffed Chicken Breast

Ingredients:

- ➤ 4 boneless, skinless chicken breasts
- ➤ 2 cups fresh spinach leaves
- ➤ 1/2 cup crumbled feta cheese
- ➤ 2 cloves garlic, minced
- ➤ 1 tablespoon olive oil
- ➤ Salt and pepper to taste

Preparation:

1) Preheat the oven to 375°F (190°C). Grease a baking dish with olive oil.

2) Using a sharp knife, cut a pocket into each chicken breast.

3) In a skillet, heat olive oil over medium heat. Add minced garlic and sauté until fragrant.

4) Add fresh spinach leaves to the skillet and cook until wilted.

Remove from heat and let cool slightly.

5) Once cooled, mix wilted spinach with crumbled feta cheese. Stuff each chicken breast with the spinach and feta mixture.

6) Place stuffed chicken breasts in the prepared baking dish. Season with salt and pepper.

7) Bake for 25-30 minutes, or until chicken is cooked through.

Number of servings: 4

Nutritional value per serving:

- Calories: 220
- Protein: 30g
- Fat: 10g
- Carbohydrates: 3g
- Fiber: 1g

Cooking time: 35 minutes

Mushroom and Spinach Quinoa Risotto

Ingredients:

- 1 cup uncooked quinoa
- 2 cups low-sodium vegetable broth
- 1 tablespoon olive oil
- 1 onion, diced
- 2 cloves garlic, minced
- 8 oz mushrooms, sliced
- 2 cups fresh spinach leaves
- 1/4 cup grated Parmesan cheese
- Salt and pepper to taste

Preparation:

1) Rinse quinoa under cold water. In a pot, bring vegetable broth to a boil. Add quinoa, reduce heat to low, cover, and simmer for 15-20 minutes, or until quinoa is cooked and liquid is absorbed.

2) In a large skillet, heat olive oil over medium heat. Add diced onion and minced garlic, and sauté until translucent.

3) Add sliced mushrooms to the skillet and cook until softened.

4) Stir cooked quinoa and fresh spinach leaves into the skillet. Cook until spinach is wilted.

5) Remove skillet from heat and stir in grated Parmesan cheese. Season with salt and pepper to taste.

Number of servings: 4

Nutritional value per serving:

- Calories: 250
- Protein: 10g
- Fat: 8g
- Carbohydrates: 35g
- Fiber: 5g

Cooking time: 25 minutes

Turkey and Vegetable Chili

Ingredients:

- 1 lb ground turkey
- 1 onion, diced
- 2 cloves garlic, minced
- 1 bell pepper, diced
- 1 zucchini, diced
- 1 can diced tomatoes
- 1 can kidney beans, drained and rinsed
- 2 cups low-sodium vegetable broth
- 1 tablespoon chili powder
- 1 teaspoon cumin
- Salt and pepper to taste

Preparation:

1) In a large pot, cook ground turkey over medium heat until browned. Add diced onion and minced garlic, and cook until softened.

2) Add diced bell pepper and zucchini to the pot, and cook until vegetables are tender.

3) Stir in diced tomatoes, kidney beans, vegetable broth, chili powder, cumin, salt, and pepper.

4) Bring chili to a boil, then reduce heat and simmer for 20-25 minutes, stirring occasionally.

5) Serve hot, garnished with your favorite toppings such as avocado, Greek yogurt, or shredded cheese.

Number of servings: 6

Nutritional value per serving:

- Calories: 280
- Protein: 20g
- Fat: 10g
- Carbohydrates: 30g
- Fiber: 8g

Cooking time: 35 minutes

Grilled Lemon Herb Shrimp Skewers

Ingredients:

- 1 lb large shrimp, peeled and deveined
- 2 tablespoons olive oil
- 2 cloves garlic, minced
- Zest and juice of 1 lemon
- 1 tablespoon fresh parsley, chopped
- 1 teaspoon dried oregano
- Salt and pepper to taste
- Lemon wedges for serving

Preparation:

1) In a bowl, toss shrimp with olive oil, minced garlic, lemon zest, lemon juice, chopped parsley, dried oregano, salt, and pepper. Let marinate for 15-20 minutes.

2) Preheat the grill or grill pan over medium-high heat. Thread shrimp onto skewers.

3) Grill shrimp skewers for 2-3 minutes per side, or until shrimp are pink and opaque.

4) Serve hot with lemon wedges for squeezing.

Number of servings: 4

Nutritional value per serving:

- Calories: 200
- Protein: 25g
- Fat: 8g
- Carbohydrates: 2g
- Fiber: 0g

Cooking time: 10 minutes

Mediterranean Chickpea Salad

Ingredients:

- 2 cans chickpeas, drained and rinsed
- 1 cucumber, diced
- 1 bell pepper, diced
- 1 red onion, diced
- 1 cup cherry tomatoes, halved
- 1/4 cup Kalamata olives, pitted and halved
- 1/4 cup crumbled feta cheese
- 2 tablespoons olive oil
- 2 tablespoons lemon juice
- 1 tablespoon fresh parsley, chopped
- Salt and pepper to taste

Preparation:

1) In a large bowl, combine chickpeas, diced cucumber, diced bell pepper, diced red onion, halved cherry tomatoes,

halved Kalamata olives, and crumbled feta cheese.

2) In a small bowl, whisk together olive oil, lemon juice, chopped parsley, salt, and pepper to make the dressing.

3) Drizzle the dressing over the salad and toss until all ingredients are evenly coated.

4) Serve chilled or at room temperature.

Number of servings: 4

Nutritional value per serving:

- Calories: 280
- Protein: 12g
- Fat: 10g
- Carbohydrates: 35g
- Fiber: 8g

Cooking time: 15 minutes

Baked Turkey Meatballs

Ingredients:

- 1 lb ground turkey
- 1/2 cup breadcrumbs
- 1/4 cup grated Parmesan cheese
- 1 egg, beaten
- 2 cloves garlic, minced
- 1 tablespoon Italian seasoning
- Salt and pepper to taste
- Marinara sauce for serving

Preparation:

1) Preheat the oven to 400°F (200°C). Line a baking sheet with parchment paper.

2) In a large bowl, combine ground turkey, breadcrumbs, grated Parmesan cheese, beaten egg, minced garlic, Italian seasoning, salt, and pepper.

3) Roll mixture into meatballs and place them on the prepared baking sheet.

4) Bake meatballs for 20-25 minutes, or until cooked through and browned.

5) Serve hot with marinara sauce.

- Calories: 230
- Protein: 25g
- Fat: 10g
- Carbohydrates: 10g
- Fiber: 2g

Sesame Ginger Tofu Stir-Fry

Ingredients:

- 1 block extra-firm tofu, pressed and cubed
- 2 tablespoons soy sauce
- 1 tablespoon sesame oil
- 1 tablespoon cornstarch
- 2 tablespoons olive oil
- 2 cups mixed vegetables (bell peppers, broccoli, snap peas)
- 2 cloves garlic, minced
- 1 tablespoon fresh ginger, minced
- 2 tablespoons hoisin sauce
- Cooked brown rice for serving

Preparation:

1) In a bowl, toss cubed tofu with soy sauce, sesame oil, and cornstarch. Let marinate for 15 minutes.

2) Heat olive oil in a large skillet or wok over medium-high heat. Add marinated tofu and cook until golden brown on all sides. Remove tofu from the skillet and set aside.

3) In the same skillet, add mixed vegetables, minced garlic, and minced ginger. Stir-fry until vegetables are tender-crisp.

4) Add cooked tofu back to the skillet and stir in hoisin sauce. Cook for an additional 2-3 minutes.

5) Serve stir-fry over cooked brown rice.

Number of servings: 4

Nutritional value per serving:

- Calories: 250
- Protein: 15g
- Fat: 12g
- Carbohydrates: 25g
- Fiber: 5g

Cooking time: 25 minutes

Pesto Zucchini Noodles with Cherry Tomatoes

Ingredients:

- 4 medium zucchini, spiralized into noodles
- 1 cup cherry tomatoes, halved
- 1/4 cup pesto sauce
- 2 tablespoons grated Parmesan cheese
- 1 tablespoon olive oil
- Salt and pepper to taste
- Fresh basil leaves for garnish

Preparation:

1) In a large skillet, heat olive oil over medium heat. Add spiralized zucchini noodles and cook for 2-3 minutes, or until just tender.

2) Add halved cherry tomatoes to the skillet and cook for an additional 1-2 minutes, until heated through.

3) Stir in pesto sauce until noodles and tomatoes are evenly coated.

4) Remove from heat and sprinkle grated Parmesan cheese over the top.

5) Garnish with fresh basil leaves before serving.

Number of servings: 4

Nutritional value per serving:

- Calories: 180
- Protein: 8g
- Fat: 10g
- Carbohydrates: 15g
- Fiber: 5g

Cooking time: 10 minutes

These main course recipes are not only delicious but also packed with essential nutrients to support bone health and overall well-being. Enjoy them as part of a balanced diet to nourish your body and promote optimal health.

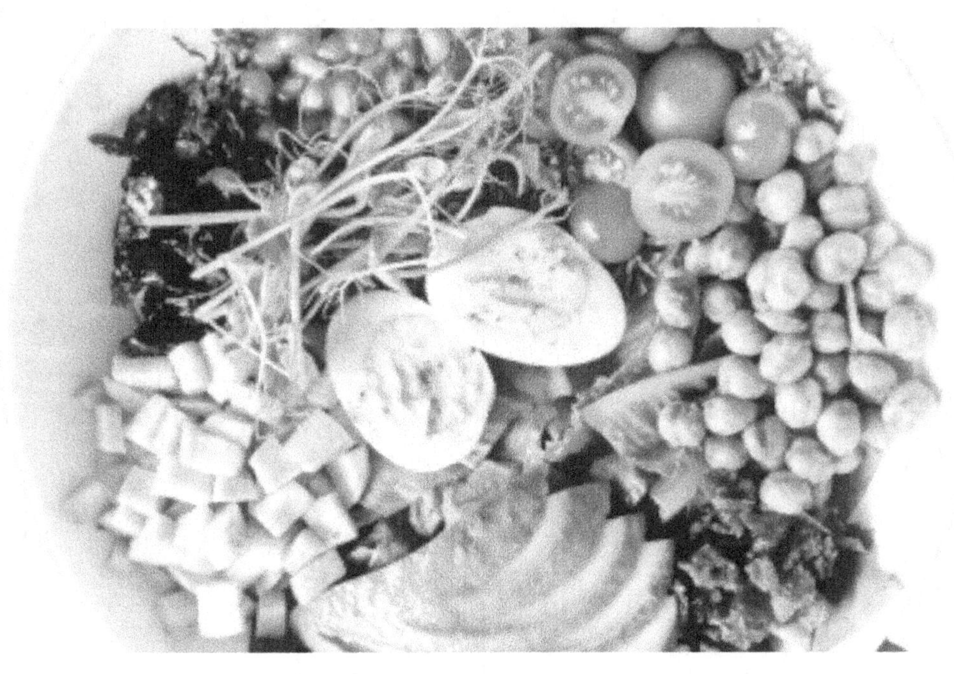

Greek Yogurt with Mixed Berries

Ingredients:

- 1/2 cup Greek yogurt (low-fat)
- 1/4 cup mixed berries (such as strawberries, blueberries, raspberries)
- 1 tablespoon chopped almonds
- 1 teaspoon honey (optional)

Preparation:

1) In a bowl, layer Greek yogurt with mixed berries.
2) Sprinkle chopped almonds on top.
3) Drizzle with honey if desired.

Number of servings: 1

Nutritional value per serving:

- Calories: 150
- Protein: 10g
- Fat: 5g
- Carbohydrates: 15g
- Fiber: 3g

Preparation time: 5 minutes

Cottage Cheese and Pineapple Skewers

Ingredients:

- 1/2 cup cottage cheese (low-fat)
- 1 cup fresh pineapple chunks
- Wooden skewers

Preparation:

1) Thread pineapple chunks onto wooden skewers.
2) Serve skewers with a side of cottage cheese for dipping.

Number of servings: 1

Nutritional value per serving:

- Calories: 120
- Protein: 10g
- Fat: 2g
- Carbohydrates: 20g
- Fiber: 2g

Preparation time: 10 minutes

Hummus with Crudité

Ingredients:

- 1/4 cup hummus
- Assorted raw vegetables (such as baby carrots, cucumber slices, bell pepper strips)

Preparation:

1) Arrange raw vegetables on a plate.
2) Serve with hummus for dipping.

Number of servings: 1

Nutritional value per serving:

- Calories: 100
- Protein: 4g
- Fat: 5g
- Carbohydrates: 10g
- Fiber: 4g

Preparation time: 5 minutes

Baked Sweet Potato Chips

Ingredients:

- 1 large sweet potato, thinly sliced
- 1 tablespoon olive oil
- Salt and pepper to taste

Preparation:

1) Preheat the oven to 375°F (190°C).
2) In a bowl, toss sweet potato slices with olive oil, salt, and pepper.
3) Arrange the slices in a single layer on a baking sheet.
4) Bake for 15-20 minutes, or until crispy and golden brown.

Number of servings: 2

Nutritional value per serving:

- Calories: 100
- Protein: 2g
- Fat: 4g
- Carbohydrates: 15g
- Fiber: 2g

Cooking time: 20 minutes

Ingredients:

- ➢ 1 cup cooked edamame (shelled)
- ➢ 1/2 cup diced cucumber
- ➢ 1/4 cup diced red bell pepper
- ➢ 2 tablespoons chopped fresh cilantro
- ➢ 1 tablespoon sesame oil
- ➢ 1 tablespoon rice vinegar
- ➢ 1 teaspoon soy sauce (low-sodium)
- ➢ Sesame seeds for garnish

Preparation:

1) In a bowl, combine cooked edamame, diced cucumber, diced red bell pepper, and chopped cilantro.
2) In a separate bowl, whisk together sesame oil, rice vinegar, and soy sauce.
3) Drizzle the dressing over the edamame salad and toss to coat.
4) Garnish with sesame seeds before serving.

Number of servings: 2

Nutritional value per serving:

- Calories: 120
- Protein: 8g
- Fat: 7g
- Carbohydrates: 10g
- Fiber: 4g

Preparation time: 10 minutes

Almond-Stuffed Dates

Ingredients:

- 4 large Medjool dates, pitted
- 4 whole almonds

Preparation:

1) Make a small slit in each date and remove the pit.
2) Stuff each date with a whole almond.
3) Serve immediately or refrigerate for later.

Number of servings: 2

Nutritional value per serving:

- Calories: 80
- Protein: 1g
- Fat: 2g
- Carbohydrates: 18g
- Fiber: 2g

Preparation time: 5 minutes

Spinach and Feta Stuffed Mushrooms

Ingredients:

- 4 large portobello mushrooms, stems removed
- 1 cup fresh spinach, chopped
- 1/4 cup crumbled feta cheese
- 1 tablespoon olive oil
- Salt and pepper to taste

Preparation:

1) Preheat the oven to 375°F (190°C).
2) Place portobello mushrooms on a baking sheet.
3) In a skillet, heat olive oil over medium heat. Add chopped spinach and cook until wilted.
4) Fill each mushroom cap with cooked spinach and crumbled feta cheese.
5) Bake for 15-20 minutes, or until mushrooms are tender.

6) Season with salt and pepper before serving.

- Calories: 80
- Protein: 4g
- Fat: 5g
- Carbohydrates: 6g
- Fiber: 2g

Tuna Cucumber Bites

Ingredients:

- 1 can (5 ounces) tuna in water, drained
- 1/4 cup Greek yogurt (low-fat)
- 1 tablespoon chopped fresh dill
- 1 cucumber, sliced into rounds
- Preparation:
- In a bowl, mix drained tuna with Greek yogurt and chopped fresh dill.
- Place cucumber rounds on a serving platter.
- Top each cucumber round with a spoonful of tuna mixture.
- Serve chilled.

- Calories: 70
- Protein: 10g
- Fat: 1g
- Carbohydrates: 5g
- Fiber: 1g

Ingredients:

- 8 cherry tomatoes
- 8 small fresh mozzarella balls
- 8 fresh basil leaves
- Balsamic glaze for drizzling
- Wooden skewers

Preparation:

1) Thread cherry tomatoes, mozzarella balls, and fresh basil leaves onto wooden skewers.
2) Arrange skewers on a serving platter.
3) Drizzle with balsamic glaze before serving.

Number of servings: 2

Nutritional value per serving:

- Calories: 100
- Protein: 6g
- Fat: 6g
- Carbohydrates: 5g
- Fiber: 1g

Preparation time: 10 minutes

Ingredients:

- 1 can chickpeas, drained and rinsed
- 2 tablespoons tahini
- 2 cloves garlic, roasted
- Juice of 1 lemon
- 2 tablespoons olive oil
- Salt and pepper to taste
- Assorted vegetable sticks (carrots, celery, bell peppers)

Preparation:

1) In a food processor, combine chickpeas, tahini, roasted garlic, lemon juice, olive oil, salt, and pepper.
2) Blend until smooth and creamy, adding water if necessary to reach desired consistency.

3) Serve hummus with assorted vegetable sticks for dipping.

- Calories: 120
- Protein: 4g
- Fat: 7g
- Carbohydrates: 12g
- Fiber: 4g

Kale Chips

Ingredients:

- ➢ 1 bunch kale, stems removed and leaves torn into bite-sized pieces
- ➢ 1 tablespoon olive oil
- ➢ 1/2 teaspoon garlic powder
- ➢ 1/2 teaspoon paprika
- ➢ Salt and pepper to taste

Preparation:

1) Preheat the oven to 300°F (150°C). Line a baking sheet with parchment paper.
2) In a large bowl, toss kale pieces with olive oil, garlic powder, paprika, salt, and pepper until evenly coated.
3) Spread kale in a single layer on the prepared baking sheet.
4) Bake for 10-15 minutes, or until kale is crispy but not burnt.

- Calories: 50
- Protein: 2g
- Fat: 3g
- Carbohydrates: 5g
- Fiber: 2g

Ingredients:

- 1 can chickpeas, drained and rinsed
- 1 roasted red pepper, peeled and seeded
- 2 tablespoons tahini
- Juice of 1 lemon
- 2 cloves garlic
- 2 tablespoons olive oil
- Salt and pepper to taste
- Whole grain crackers for serving

Preparation:

1) In a food processor, combine chickpeas, roasted red pepper, tahini, lemon juice, garlic, olive oil, salt, and pepper.
2) Blend until smooth and creamy, adding water if necessary to reach desired consistency.
3) Serve hummus with whole grain crackers for dipping.

Number of servings: 4

Nutritional value per serving:

- Calories: 120
- Protein: 3g
- Fat: 7g
- Carbohydrates: 12g
- Fiber: 3g

Preparation time: 15 minutes

These snacks and sides recipes are not only delicious and satisfying but also packed with essential nutrients to support bone health and overall well-being. Enjoying a variety of nutrient-rich foods as part of a balanced diet is key to managing and preventing osteoporosis while promoting optimal health.

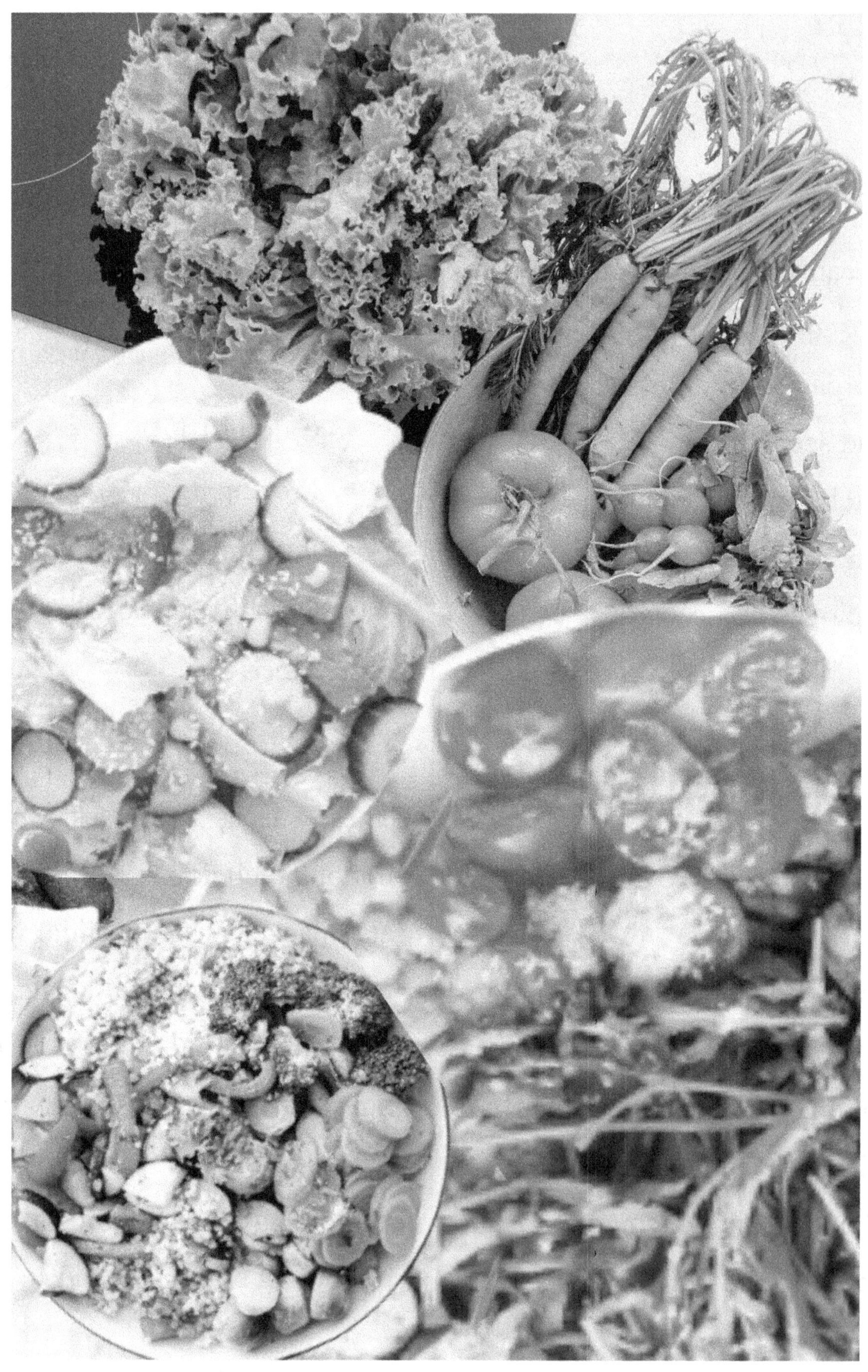

Exercise for Strong Bones:

Regular exercise is crucial for maintaining strong and healthy bones. Weight-bearing and resistance exercises are particularly beneficial for bone health. Weight-bearing exercises involve activities that make you move against gravity while staying upright, such as walking, jogging, hiking, dancing, and stair climbing. These activities help to stimulate bone formation and increase bone density.

Resistance exercises, on the other hand, involve using weights or resistance bands to strengthen muscles and bones. Examples of resistance exercises include weightlifting, using resistance bands, and bodyweight exercises like squats, lunges, and push-ups. These exercises place stress on the bones, stimulating them to grow stronger and denser over time.

It's important to engage in a variety of exercises that target different muscle groups and bone-loading patterns to promote overall bone health. Aim for at least 30 minutes of weight-bearing or resistance exercise most days of the week, in addition to incorporating flexibility and balance exercises for overall fitness.

Sunlight and Vitamin D:

Sunlight exposure is essential for the body to produce vitamin D, which plays a crucial role in bone health.

When sunlight hits the skin, it triggers the production of vitamin D in the body.

Vitamin D helps the body absorb calcium, a key mineral for building and maintaining strong bones. Without adequate vitamin D, the body may struggle to absorb calcium efficiently, leading to weakened bones and an increased risk of fractures.

To maintain optimal vitamin D levels, aim for regular, moderate sun exposure while taking precautions to protect your skin from sunburn and skin damage. Spending about 10 to 30 minutes outdoors in the sun without sunscreen several times a week, particularly during the midday hours when the sun is strongest, can help your body produce an adequate amount of vitamin D. However, factors such as skin pigmentation,

geographic location, season, and use of sunscreen can affect vitamin D synthesis.

In addition to sunlight exposure, it's important to include dietary sources of vitamin D in your diet, such as fatty fish (salmon, mackerel, tuna), egg yolks, fortified dairy products, and fortified plant-based milk alternatives. If you have difficulty obtaining enough vitamin D from sunlight and diet alone, your healthcare provider may recommend vitamin D supplements to ensure you meet your daily needs.

Managing Medications and Supplements:

Certain medications and supplements can impact bone health, either positively or negatively. It's important to be aware of the effects of these substances and to work with your healthcare provider to manage them effectively.

Some medications, such as corticosteroids (used to treat conditions like asthma, rheumatoid arthritis, and lupus), can weaken bones over time by interfering with the bone remodeling process and reducing calcium absorption. If you're taking long-term corticosteroids, your healthcare provider may recommend strategies to minimize bone loss, such as calcium and vitamin D supplementation, weight-bearing exercise, and bone density monitoring.

Conversely, certain medications and supplements can support bone health. For example, calcium and vitamin D supplements are often recommended for individuals at risk of osteoporosis or those who have difficulty obtaining enough of these nutrients from their diet or sunlight exposure alone. Other supplements, such as magnesium, vitamin K, and collagen, may also play a role in bone health and may be beneficial when taken as part of a comprehensive approach to bone health.

It's important to discuss any medications or supplements you're taking with your healthcare provider to ensure they are appropriate for your individual needs and to monitor their effects on your bone health over time. Your healthcare provider can offer personalized recommendations based on your medical history, risk factors, and lifestyle factors to support optimal bone health.

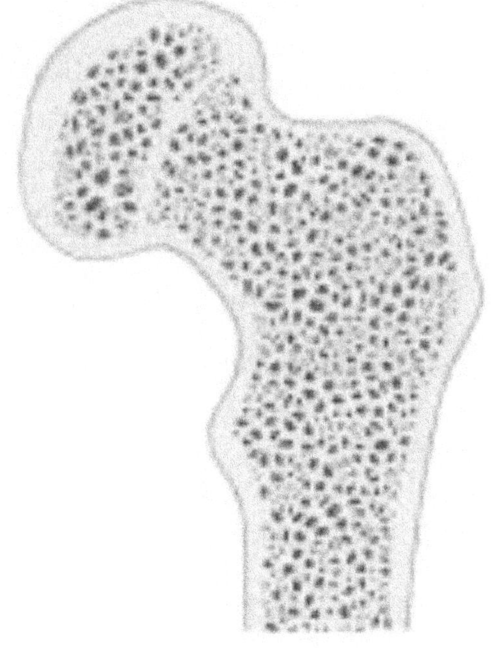

OSTEOPOROSIS
HEALTHY BONE

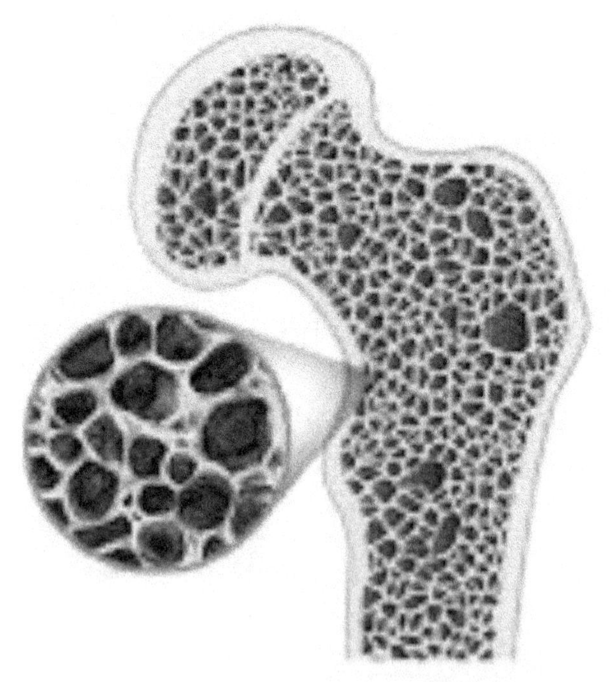

OSTEOPOROSIS

1. Dealing with Bone Fractures:

Bone fractures are a common concern for individuals with osteoporosis due to weakened bones. Dealing with bone fractures involves prompt treatment and rehabilitation to promote healing and prevent further complications. Here are some key steps in managing bone fractures:

I. **Seek immediate medical attention:** If you suspect you have sustained a bone fracture, seek medical attention promptly. Your healthcare provider will perform diagnostic tests, such as X-rays, to assess the extent of the fracture and determine the appropriate treatment.

II. **Immobilization:** Depending on the severity and location of the fracture, immobilization may be necessary to allow the bone to heal properly. This may involve the use of casts, splints, or braces to stabilize the affected area.

III. **Pain management:** Fractures can be painful, so pain management strategies may be recommended to help alleviate discomfort. This may include over-the-counter or prescription pain medications, as well as ice packs or heat therapy to reduce inflammation and pain.

IV. **Rehabilitation:** Once the fracture begins to heal, rehabilitation exercises may be prescribed to restore strength, flexibility, and mobility in the affected area. Physical therapy can help prevent muscle atrophy and improve function.

V. **Fall prevention:** Taking steps to prevent future falls is crucial for individuals with osteoporosis to reduce the risk of sustaining additional fractures. This may involve modifying the home environment to remove hazards, wearing supportive footwear, using assistive devices such as canes or walkers, and participating in balance and strength training exercises.

Pain management is an important aspect of managing osteoporosis symptoms, particularly for individuals who experience chronic pain or discomfort. Here are some pain management techniques that may be helpful:

I. **Medications:** Over-the-counter or prescription pain medications, such as nonsteroidal anti-inflammatory drugs (NSAIDs), acetaminophen, or opioids, may be prescribed to help alleviate pain associated with osteoporosis.

II. **Physical therapy:** Physical therapy can be beneficial for individuals with osteoporosis-related pain by improving strength, flexibility, and posture, as well as addressing any underlying muscle imbalances or weaknesses.

III. **Hot and cold therapy:** Applying heat packs or ice packs to the affected area can help reduce inflammation and relieve pain. Heat therapy can help relax muscles and increase blood flow, while cold therapy can numb the area and reduce swelling.

IV. **Relaxation techniques:** Stress and tension can exacerbate pain, so relaxation techniques such as deep breathing exercises, meditation, or guided imagery may help reduce pain and promote relaxation.

V. **Lifestyle modifications:** Making lifestyle changes such as maintaining a healthy weight, practicing good posture, staying physically active, and getting an adequate amount of sleep can all contribute to managing pain associated with osteoporosis.

3. Fall Prevention Tips:

Preventing falls is crucial for individuals with osteoporosis to reduce the risk of fractures and other injuries. Here are some fall prevention tips:

I. **Maintain a safe home environment:** Remove tripping hazards such as loose rugs, electrical cords, and clutter from walkways. Install handrails on staircases and grab bars in bathrooms to provide support and stability.

II. **Use assistive devices:** Consider using assistive devices such as canes, walkers, or walking poles to improve balance and reduce the risk of falls, especially when navigating uneven terrain or unfamiliar environments.

III. **Wear supportive footwear:** Choose shoes with non-slip soles and good arch support to provide stability and reduce the risk of slipping or tripping.

IV. **Stay physically active:** Engage in regular exercise to improve strength, balance, and coordination. Activities such as walking, tai chi, yoga, and strength training can help reduce the risk of falls by improving muscle strength and flexibility.

V. **Have regular vision and hearing checks:** Poor vision or hearing can increase the risk of falls, so it's important to have regular check-ups and address any vision or hearing issues promptly.

VI. **Review medications:** Some medications can cause dizziness or drowsiness, increasing the risk of falls. Review your medications with your healthcare provider to identify any potential side effects and make adjustments as needed.

By implementing these strategies, you can effectively manage symptoms, reduce the risk of fractures, and improve overall quality of life.

Holistic Approaches to Osteoporosis Care:

Stress Reduction and Mental Health:

Stress reduction and mental health play important roles in overall well-being and can impact bone health in individuals with osteoporosis. Chronic stress can lead to increased levels of cortisol, a hormone that can contribute to bone loss over time. Additionally, stress can lead to unhealthy coping behaviors such as poor diet, lack of exercise, and inadequate sleep, all of which can negatively affect bone health.

Implementing stress reduction techniques can help mitigate the impact of stress on bone health and promote overall wellness. These techniques may include:

Mindfulness and meditation: Practicing mindfulness techniques such as deep breathing exercises, meditation, and progressive muscle relaxation can help reduce stress levels and promote relaxation.

Physical activity: Engaging in regular physical activity, such as walking, yoga, or tai chi, can help alleviate stress and improve mood by releasing endorphins, the body's natural mood lifters.

Social support: Maintaining strong social connections and seeking support from friends, family, or support groups can provide emotional support and reduce feelings of isolation and stress.

Counseling or therapy: Talking to a mental health professional can provide strategies for coping with stress, anxiety, or depression and improve overall mental well-being.

By prioritizing stress reduction and mental health, individuals with osteoporosis can enhance their overall quality of life and support their bone health.

Sleep Hygiene and Bone Health:

Sleep plays a crucial role in bone health, as it is during sleep that the body undergoes important repair and regeneration processes. Poor sleep quality or inadequate sleep duration can interfere with these processes and negatively impact bone health over time.

Here are some tips for improving sleep hygiene and promoting bone health:

Maintain a consistent sleep schedule: Going to bed and waking up at the same time each day helps regulate your body's internal clock and promote better sleep quality.

Create a relaxing bedtime routine: Engage in relaxing activities such as reading, taking a warm bath, or practicing relaxation techniques before bedtime to signal to your body that it's time to wind down.

Create a conducive sleep environment: Ensure your bedroom is quiet, dark, and cool, and invest in a comfortable mattress and pillows to support restful sleep.

Limit screen time before bed: Exposure to blue light from electronic devices such as smartphones, tablets, and computers can interfere with sleep patterns. Limit screen time at least an hour before bedtime.

Avoid stimulants: Limit consumption of caffeine, nicotine, and alcohol, especially in the hours leading up to bedtime, as they can disrupt sleep patterns.

Manage stress: Practice stress reduction techniques such as mindfulness, meditation, or deep breathing exercises to help relax the mind and body before bedtime.

By prioritizing sleep hygiene and ensuring adequate rest, individuals with osteoporosis can support their body's natural repair processes and promote overall bone health.

Complementary Therapies and Their Efficacy:

Complementary therapies, also known as alternative or integrative therapies, encompass a wide range of practices and treatments that are used alongside conventional medical care to promote health and well-being. While research on the efficacy of complementary therapies for osteoporosis specifically is limited, some therapies may offer potential benefits in supporting bone health and overall wellness.

Some complementary therapies that individuals with osteoporosis may consider include:

Acupuncture: Acupuncture is a traditional Chinese medicine practice that involves inserting thin needles into specific points on the body to stimulate energy flow and promote healing. Some studies suggest that acupuncture may help reduce pain and improve quality of life in individuals with osteoporosis-related pain.

Herbal supplements: Certain herbal supplements, such as red clover, black cohosh, and horsetail, have been studied for their potential benefits in promoting bone health. However, more research is needed to determine their safety and efficacy in managing osteoporosis.

Massage therapy: Massage therapy involves manipulating the soft tissues of the body to promote relaxation and relieve muscle tension. While massage therapy may not directly impact bone density, it can help alleviate muscle pain and stiffness associated with osteoporosis and improve overall quality of life.

Tai chi: Tai chi is a mind-body practice that combines gentle movements, deep breathing, and meditation to promote relaxation, balance, and flexibility. Some research suggests that tai chi may help improve balance, reduce falls, and enhance quality of life in individuals with osteoporosis.

It's important to approach complementary therapies with caution and discuss their use with a healthcare provider, especially if you have underlying health conditions or are taking medications. While some complementary therapies may offer potential benefits in managing osteoporosis symptoms and promoting overall wellness, they should not replace conventional medical care or treatment. Additionally, more research is needed to fully understand the efficacy and safety of these therapies for individuals with osteoporosis.

In conclusion, the "Osteoporosis Diet Cookbook for Seniors" serves as a comprehensive guide to understanding and managing osteoporosis through nutrition and lifestyle choices. Throughout this cookbook, we have explored the fundamentals of osteoporosis, including its causes, symptoms, risk factors, and the crucial role that diet plays in prevention and management. From nutrient-rich breakfasts to wholesome lunches and delicious snacks, each recipe has been thoughtfully crafted to provide essential nutrients such as calcium, vitamin D, protein, magnesium, and vitamin K—key components of a bone-healthy diet.

Moreover, we have delved into holistic approaches to osteoporosis care, recognizing the importance of stress reduction, quality sleep, and complementary therapies in supporting bone health and overall well-being. By addressing these aspects of health in conjunction with dietary interventions, individuals with osteoporosis can optimize their treatment outcomes and improve their quality of life.

It is important to emphasize that adopting a bone-healthy diet is not just about managing a condition—it is about embracing a lifestyle that promotes vitality, strength, and longevity. By nourishing our bodies with wholesome foods and engaging in regular physical activity, we empower ourselves to take control of our health and reduce the risk of fractures and other complications associated with osteoporosis.

To the readers of this cookbook, I offer a special motivation: envision a future filled with vitality and independence, where you can enjoy life to the fullest without the limitations imposed by osteoporosis. By incorporating the recipes and strategies outlined in this cookbook into your daily routine, you are investing in your health and well-being, laying the foundation for a stronger, healthier future.

Remember, small changes can lead to significant improvements over time. Whether you are newly diagnosed with osteoporosis or have been managing the condition for years, there is always room for growth and improvement. With dedication, perseverance, and the support of loved ones and healthcare professionals, you can overcome the challenges posed by osteoporosis and live a fulfilling, active life.

As you embark on this journey towards better bone health, I encourage you to approach it with an open mind and a sense of empowerment. You have the ability to make positive changes in your life, starting with the food choices you make each day. Together, let us embrace the power of nutrition to nourish our bones, strengthen our bodies, and live life to the fullest.

WEEKLY MEAL PLANNER

MONDAY

BREAKFAST _______________________

LUNCH _______________________

SNACKS _______________________

DINNER _______________________

TUESDAY

BREAKFAST _______________________

LUNCH _______________________

SNACKS _______________________

DINNER _______________________

WEDNESDAY

BREAKFAST _______________________

LUNCH _______________________

SNACKS _______________________

DINNER _______________________

THURSDAY

BREAKFAST _______________________

LUNCH _______________________

SNACKS _______________________

DINNER _______________________

FRIDAY

BREAKFAST _______________________

LUNCH _______________________

SNACKS _______________________

DINNER _______________________

SATURDAY

BREAKFAST _______________________

LUNCH _______________________

SNACKS _______________________

DINNER _______________________

SUNDAY

BREAKFAST _______________________

LUNCH _______________________

SNACKS _______________________

DINNER _______________________

NOTES

____

____

____

____

WEEKLY MEAL PLANNER

MONDAY

BREAKFAST ___________________

LUNCH ___________________

SNACKS ___________________

DINNER ___________________

TUESDAY

BREAKFAST ___________________

LUNCH ___________________

SNACKS ___________________

DINNER ___________________

WEDNESDAY

BREAKFAST ___________________

LUNCH ___________________

SNACKS ___________________

DINNER ___________________

THURSDAY

BREAKFAST ___________________

LUNCH ___________________

SNACKS ___________________

DINNER ___________________

FRIDAY

BREAKFAST ___________________

LUNCH ___________________

SNACKS ___________________

DINNER ___________________

SATURDAY

BREAKFAST ___________________

LUNCH ___________________

SNACKS ___________________

DINNER ___________________

SUNDAY

BREAKFAST ___________________

LUNCH ___________________

SNACKS ___________________

DINNER ___________________

NOTES

____

____

____

____

WEEKLY MEAL PLANNER

MONDAY

BREAKFAST _______________________

LUNCH _______________________

SNACKS _______________________

DINNER _______________________

TUESDAY

BREAKFAST _______________________

LUNCH _______________________

SNACKS _______________________

DINNER _______________________

WEDNESDAY

BREAKFAST _______________________

LUNCH _______________________

SNACKS _______________________

DINNER _______________________

THURSDAY

BREAKFAST _______________________

LUNCH _______________________

SNACKS _______________________

DINNER _______________________

FRIDAY

BREAKFAST _______________________

LUNCH _______________________

SNACKS _______________________

DINNER _______________________

SATURDAY

BREAKFAST _______________________

LUNCH _______________________

SNACKS _______________________

DINNER _______________________

SUNDAY

BREAKFAST _______________________

LUNCH _______________________

SNACKS _______________________

DINNER _______________________

NOTES

____

____

____

WEEKLY MEAL PLANNER

MONDAY

BREAKFAST _______________________

LUNCH _______________________

SNACKS _______________________

DINNER _______________________

TUESDAY

BREAKFAST _______________________

LUNCH _______________________

SNACKS _______________________

DINNER _______________________

WEDNESDAY

BREAKFAST _______________________

LUNCH _______________________

SNACKS _______________________

DINNER _______________________

THURSDAY

BREAKFAST _______________________

LUNCH _______________________

SNACKS _______________________

DINNER _______________________

FRIDAY

BREAKFAST _______________________

LUNCH _______________________

SNACKS _______________________

DINNER _______________________

SATURDAY

BREAKFAST _______________________

LUNCH _______________________

SNACKS _______________________

DINNER _______________________

SUNDAY

BREAKFAST _______________________

LUNCH _______________________

SNACKS _______________________

DINNER _______________________

NOTES

____

____

____

____

WEEKLY MEAL PLANNER

MONDAY

BREAKFAST _______________________

LUNCH _______________________

SNACKS _______________________

DINNER _______________________

TUESDAY

BREAKFAST _______________________

LUNCH _______________________

SNACKS _______________________

DINNER _______________________

WEDNESDAY

BREAKFAST _______________________

LUNCH _______________________

SNACKS _______________________

DINNER _______________________

THURSDAY

BREAKFAST _______________________

LUNCH _______________________

SNACKS _______________________

DINNER _______________________

FRIDAY

BREAKFAST _______________________

LUNCH _______________________

SNACKS _______________________

DINNER _______________________

SATURDAY

BREAKFAST _______________________

LUNCH _______________________

SNACKS _______________________

DINNER _______________________

SUNDAY

BREAKFAST _______________________

LUNCH _______________________

SNACKS _______________________

DINNER _______________________

NOTES

____

____

____

____

WEEKLY MEAL PLANNER

MONDAY

BREAKFAST ___________________

LUNCH ___________________

SNACKS ___________________

DINNER ___________________

TUESDAY

BREAKFAST ___________________

LUNCH ___________________

SNACKS ___________________

DINNER ___________________

WEDNESDAY

BREAKFAST ___________________

LUNCH ___________________

SNACKS ___________________

DINNER ___________________

THURSDAY

BREAKFAST ___________________

LUNCH ___________________

SNACKS ___________________

DINNER ___________________

FRIDAY

BREAKFAST ___________________

LUNCH ___________________

SNACKS ___________________

DINNER ___________________

SATURDAY

BREAKFAST ___________________

LUNCH ___________________

SNACKS ___________________

DINNER ___________________

SUNDAY

BREAKFAST ___________________

LUNCH ___________________

SNACKS ___________________

DINNER ___________________

NOTES

____

____

____

____

WEEKLY MEAL PLANNER

MONDAY

BREAKFAST _______________________

LUNCH _______________________

SNACKS _______________________

DINNER _______________________

TUESDAY

BREAKFAST _______________________

LUNCH _______________________

SNACKS _______________________

DINNER _______________________

WEDNESDAY

BREAKFAST _______________________

LUNCH _______________________

SNACKS _______________________

DINNER _______________________

THURSDAY

BREAKFAST _______________________

LUNCH _______________________

SNACKS _______________________

DINNER _______________________

FRIDAY

BREAKFAST _______________________

LUNCH _______________________

SNACKS _______________________

DINNER _______________________

SATURDAY

BREAKFAST _______________________

LUNCH _______________________

SNACKS _______________________

DINNER _______________________

SUNDAY

BREAKFAST _______________________

LUNCH _______________________

SNACKS _______________________

DINNER _______________________

NOTES

____

____

____

____

WEEKLY MEAL PLANNER

<table>
<tr><td>

MONDAY

BREAKFAST _______________

LUNCH _______________

SNACKS _______________

DINNER _______________

</td><td>

TUESDAY

BREAKFAST _______________

LUNCH _______________

SNACKS _______________

DINNER _______________

</td></tr>
<tr><td>

WEDNESDAY

BREAKFAST _______________

LUNCH _______________

SNACKS _______________

DINNER _______________

</td><td>

THURSDAY

BREAKFAST _______________

LUNCH _______________

SNACKS _______________

DINNER _______________

</td></tr>
<tr><td>

FRIDAY

BREAKFAST _______________

LUNCH _______________

SNACKS _______________

DINNER _______________

</td><td>

SATURDAY

BREAKFAST _______________

LUNCH _______________

SNACKS _______________

DINNER _______________

</td></tr>
<tr><td>

SUNDAY

BREAKFAST _______________

LUNCH _______________

SNACKS _______________

DINNER _______________

</td><td>

NOTES

____

____

____

____

</td></tr>
</table>

WEEKLY MEAL PLANNER

MONDAY

BREAKFAST ___________________

LUNCH ___________________

SNACKS ___________________

DINNER ___________________

TUESDAY

BREAKFAST ___________________

LUNCH ___________________

SNACKS ___________________

DINNER ___________________

WEDNESDAY

BREAKFAST ___________________

LUNCH ___________________

SNACKS ___________________

DINNER ___________________

THURSDAY

BREAKFAST ___________________

LUNCH ___________________

SNACKS ___________________

DINNER ___________________

FRIDAY

BREAKFAST ___________________

LUNCH ___________________

SNACKS ___________________

DINNER ___________________

SATURDAY

BREAKFAST ___________________

LUNCH ___________________

SNACKS ___________________

DINNER ___________________

SUNDAY

BREAKFAST ___________________

LUNCH ___________________

SNACKS ___________________

DINNER ___________________

NOTES

____

____

____

____

WEEKLY MEAL PLANNER

MONDAY

BREAKFAST _______________

LUNCH _______________

SNACKS _______________

DINNER _______________

TUESDAY

BREAKFAST _______________

LUNCH _______________

SNACKS _______________

DINNER _______________

WEDNESDAY

BREAKFAST _______________

LUNCH _______________

SNACKS _______________

DINNER _______________

THURSDAY

BREAKFAST _______________

LUNCH _______________

SNACKS _______________

DINNER _______________

FRIDAY

BREAKFAST _______________

LUNCH _______________

SNACKS _______________

DINNER _______________

SATURDAY

BREAKFAST _______________

LUNCH _______________

SNACKS _______________

DINNER _______________

SUNDAY

BREAKFAST _______________

LUNCH _______________

SNACKS _______________

DINNER _______________

NOTES

____

____

____

____

WEEKLY MEAL PLANNER

MONDAY

BREAKFAST _______________________

LUNCH _______________________

SNACKS _______________________

DINNER _______________________

TUESDAY

BREAKFAST _______________________

LUNCH _______________________

SNACKS _______________________

DINNER _______________________

WEDNESDAY

BREAKFAST _______________________

LUNCH _______________________

SNACKS _______________________

DINNER _______________________

THURSDAY

BREAKFAST _______________________

LUNCH _______________________

SNACKS _______________________

DINNER _______________________

FRIDAY

BREAKFAST _______________________

LUNCH _______________________

SNACKS _______________________

DINNER _______________________

SATURDAY

BREAKFAST _______________________

LUNCH _______________________

SNACKS _______________________

DINNER _______________________

SUNDAY

BREAKFAST _______________________

LUNCH _______________________

SNACKS _______________________

DINNER _______________________

NOTES

____

____

____

____

WEEKLY MEAL PLANNER

MONDAY

BREAKFAST _______________________

LUNCH _______________________

SNACKS _______________________

DINNER _______________________

TUESDAY

BREAKFAST _______________________

LUNCH _______________________

SNACKS _______________________

DINNER _______________________

WEDNESDAY

BREAKFAST _______________________

LUNCH _______________________

SNACKS _______________________

DINNER _______________________

THURSDAY

BREAKFAST _______________________

LUNCH _______________________

SNACKS _______________________

DINNER _______________________

FRIDAY

BREAKFAST _______________________

LUNCH _______________________

SNACKS _______________________

DINNER _______________________

SATURDAY

BREAKFAST _______________________

LUNCH _______________________

SNACKS _______________________

DINNER _______________________

SUNDAY

BREAKFAST _______________________

LUNCH _______________________

SNACKS _______________________

DINNER _______________________

NOTES

____

____

____

____

WEEKLY MEAL PLANNER

MONDAY

BREAKFAST _______________________

LUNCH _______________________

SNACKS _______________________

DINNER _______________________

TUESDAY

BREAKFAST _______________________

LUNCH _______________________

SNACKS _______________________

DINNER _______________________

WEDNESDAY

BREAKFAST _______________________

LUNCH _______________________

SNACKS _______________________

DINNER _______________________

THURSDAY

BREAKFAST _______________________

LUNCH _______________________

SNACKS _______________________

DINNER _______________________

FRIDAY

BREAKFAST _______________________

LUNCH _______________________

SNACKS _______________________

DINNER _______________________

SATURDAY

BREAKFAST _______________________

LUNCH _______________________

SNACKS _______________________

DINNER _______________________

SUNDAY

BREAKFAST _______________________

LUNCH _______________________

SNACKS _______________________

DINNER _______________________

NOTES

____

____

____

____

WEEKLY MEAL PLANNER

MONDAY

BREAKFAST ___________________

LUNCH ___________________

SNACKS ___________________

DINNER ___________________

TUESDAY

BREAKFAST ___________________

LUNCH ___________________

SNACKS ___________________

DINNER ___________________

WEDNESDAY

BREAKFAST ___________________

LUNCH ___________________

SNACKS ___________________

DINNER ___________________

THURSDAY

BREAKFAST ___________________

LUNCH ___________________

SNACKS ___________________

DINNER ___________________

FRIDAY

BREAKFAST ___________________

LUNCH ___________________

SNACKS ___________________

DINNER ___________________

SATURDAY

BREAKFAST ___________________

LUNCH ___________________

SNACKS ___________________

DINNER ___________________

SUNDAY

BREAKFAST ___________________

LUNCH ___________________

SNACKS ___________________

DINNER ___________________

NOTES

____

____

____

____

WEEKLY MEAL PLANNER

MONDAY

BREAKFAST ___________________

LUNCH ___________________

SNACKS ___________________

DINNER ___________________

TUESDAY

BREAKFAST ___________________

LUNCH ___________________

SNACKS ___________________

DINNER ___________________

WEDNESDAY

BREAKFAST ___________________

LUNCH ___________________

SNACKS ___________________

DINNER ___________________

THURSDAY

BREAKFAST ___________________

LUNCH ___________________

SNACKS ___________________

DINNER ___________________

FRIDAY

BREAKFAST ___________________

LUNCH ___________________

SNACKS ___________________

DINNER ___________________

SATURDAY

BREAKFAST ___________________

LUNCH ___________________

SNACKS ___________________

DINNER ___________________

SUNDAY

BREAKFAST ___________________

LUNCH ___________________

SNACKS ___________________

DINNER ___________________

NOTES

____

____

____

____

WEEKLY MEAL PLANNER

MONDAY

BREAKFAST _______________________

LUNCH _______________________

SNACKS _______________________

DINNER _______________________

TUESDAY

BREAKFAST _______________________

LUNCH _______________________

SNACKS _______________________

DINNER _______________________

WEDNESDAY

BREAKFAST _______________________

LUNCH _______________________

SNACKS _______________________

DINNER _______________________

THURSDAY

BREAKFAST _______________________

LUNCH _______________________

SNACKS _______________________

DINNER _______________________

FRIDAY

BREAKFAST _______________________

LUNCH _______________________

SNACKS _______________________

DINNER _______________________

SATURDAY

BREAKFAST _______________________

LUNCH _______________________

SNACKS _______________________

DINNER _______________________

SUNDAY

BREAKFAST _______________________

LUNCH _______________________

SNACKS _______________________

DINNER _______________________

NOTES

____

____

____

____

WEEKLY MEAL PLANNER

MONDAY

BREAKFAST _______________________

LUNCH _______________________

SNACKS _______________________

DINNER _______________________

TUESDAY

BREAKFAST _______________________

LUNCH _______________________

SNACKS _______________________

DINNER _______________________

WEDNESDAY

BREAKFAST _______________________

LUNCH _______________________

SNACKS _______________________

DINNER _______________________

THURSDAY

BREAKFAST _______________________

LUNCH _______________________

SNACKS _______________________

DINNER _______________________

FRIDAY

BREAKFAST _______________________

LUNCH _______________________

SNACKS _______________________

DINNER _______________________

SATURDAY

BREAKFAST _______________________

LUNCH _______________________

SNACKS _______________________

DINNER _______________________

SUNDAY

BREAKFAST _______________________

LUNCH _______________________

SNACKS _______________________

DINNER _______________________

NOTES

____

____

____

____

WEEKLY MEAL PLANNER

MONDAY

BREAKFAST _______________________

LUNCH _______________________

SNACKS _______________________

DINNER _______________________

TUESDAY

BREAKFAST _______________________

LUNCH _______________________

SNACKS _______________________

DINNER _______________________

WEDNESDAY

BREAKFAST _______________________

LUNCH _______________________

SNACKS _______________________

DINNER _______________________

THURSDAY

BREAKFAST _______________________

LUNCH _______________________

SNACKS _______________________

DINNER _______________________

FRIDAY

BREAKFAST _______________________

LUNCH _______________________

SNACKS _______________________

DINNER _______________________

SATURDAY

BREAKFAST _______________________

LUNCH _______________________

SNACKS _______________________

DINNER _______________________

SUNDAY

BREAKFAST _______________________

LUNCH _______________________

SNACKS _______________________

DINNER _______________________

NOTES

____

____

____

____